Intellectual Disability Psychiatry

Intellectual Disability Psychiatry

A practical handbook

Editors

Angela Hassiotis
Senior Lecturer
Department of Mental Health Sciences
University College London
UK

Diana Andrea Barron
Clinical Research Fellow
Department of Mental Health Sciences
University College London
UK

Ian Hall
Consultant Psychiatrist
East London NHS Foundation Trust
UK

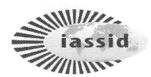

Endorsed by the International Association for
the Scientific Study of Intellectual Disabilities

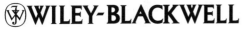

A John Wiley & Sons, Ltd., Publication

Other Wiley Editorial Offices

John Wiley & Sons Inc., 111 River Street, Hoboken, NJ 07030, USA

Jossey-Bass, 989 Market Street, San Francisco, CA 94103-1741, USA

Wiley-VCH Verlag GmbH, Boschstr. 12, D-69469 Weinheim, Germany

John Wiley & Sons Australia Ltd, 33 Park Road, Milton, Queensland 4064, Australia

John Wiley & Sons (Asia) Pte Ltd, 2 Clementi Loop #02-01, Jin Xing Distripark, Singapore 129809

John Wiley & Sons Canada Ltd, 6045 Freemont Blvd, Mississauga, Ontario, L5R 4J3, Canada

Wiley also publishes its books in a variety of electronic formats. Some content that appears in print may not be
available in electronic books.

Library of Congress Cataloguing-in-Publication Data
Intellectual disability psychiatry : a practical handbook / editors, Angela Hassiotis, Diana Andrea Barron, Ian Hall.
  p. ; cm.
  Includes bibliographical references and index.
  ISBN 978-0-470-74251-8 (alk. paper)
  1. People with mental disabilities – Mental health.   I. Hassiotis, Angela. II. Barron, Diana Andrea. III. Hall, Ian P.
  [DNLM: 1.   Mental Disorders – psychology. 2.   Mental Health Services. 3.   Mentally Disabled
Persons – psychology.   WM 140 I606 2009]
  RC570.2.I65 2009
  616.89 – dc22

                                                                                        2009024882

British Library Cataloguing in Publication Data

A catalogue record for this book is available from the British Library

ISBN 9780470742518

Typeset in 10.5/13 pt Bembo by Laserwords Private Limited, Chennai, India

This book is printed on acid-free paper

Cover Illustration by Manzur Sobhan

Contents

List of Contributors

Afia Ali
East London NHS Foundation Trust
London E1 4DG
UK

Diana Andrea Barron
UCL Department of Mental Health
   Sciences
London W1W 7EJ
UK

Elspeth Bradley
Surrey Place Centre
Department of Psychiatry
Toronto ON M5T 1R8
Canada

Basil Cardoza
ABM University NHS Trust
Learning Disability Directorate
Cardiff CF5 5WF
UK

Peter Carpenter
Kingswood CLDT
Bristol BS15 8PQ
UK

Anna Cooper
Division of Community Based Sciences
University of Glasgow
Psychological Medicine Academic
   Centre
Gartnavel Royal Hospital
1055 Great Western road
Glasgow G12 0XH
UK

Shoumitro Deb
Department of Psychiatry
University of Birmingham
Edgbaston
Birmingham B15 2TT
UK

Philip Dodd
St Michael's House
Ballymun
Dublin 9
Ireland

Rebecca Goody
Cornwall Partnership NHS Trust
Bodmin PL31 1AQ
UK

Ian Hall
East London NHS Foundation Trust
London E1 4DG
UK

Angela Hassiotis
UCL Department of Mental Health
    Sciences
London W1W 7EJ
UK

William Howie
Assessment and Intervention Team
South West London and St George's
    Mental Health NHS Trust
London
UK

Michael Kerr
Welsh Centre for Learning Disabilities
Cardiff CF14 3BG
UK

Andrew Levitas
Department of Psychiatry
University of Medicine and Dentistry
    New Jersey UMDNJ/SOM
Stratford NJ 08084
USA

Shirley McMillan
Surrey Place Centre
Toronto, Ontario M5S 2C2
Canada

Helen Miller
Adult Team National Deaf Services
South West London and St George's
    Mental Health Services NHS Trust
London SW12 9HW
UK

Deirdre O'Brady
East London NHS Foundation Trust
London E1 4DG
UK

Katrina Scior
Research Department of Clinical,
    Educational and Health Psychology
London WC1E 6BT
UK

Neill Simpson
East Dunbartonshire JLDT
Kirkintilloch G66 1XQ
UK

Amanda Sinai
Camden Learning Disabilities Service
London NW1 7JR
UK

David Smith
CAMHS
South West London and St George's
    Mental Health NHS Trust
London
UK

Andre Strydom
Department of Mental Health
    Sciences
Hampstead Campus
London NW3 2PF
UK

Jennifer Torr
Centre for Developmental Health
    Victoria
Monash University
Notting Hill
Australia

Petricia Noonan Walsh
Centre for Disability Studies
University College Dublin
Belfield, Dublin 4
Ireland

Emma Whicher
Adult Team National Deaf Services
South West London and St George's
    Mental Health Services NHS Trust
London SW12 9HW
UK

Emma Winn
Camden Learning Disabilities Service
London NW1 7JR
UK

Evan Yacoub
East London NHS Foundation Trust
London E1 4DG
UK

Foreword

People with intellectual disabilities are among the most complex and most rewarding of people to work with and the changes in attitudes, in services and in working practices that have occurred in this field in the UK and in some other parts of the world have been truly remarkable. Central to such changes has been the recognition of the importance of respect for the human rights of people with intellectual disabilities, as exemplified by the recent UN Convention on the Rights of Persons with Disabilities, together with an understanding that people with intellectual disabilities vary considerably in the nature and extent of their needs and in their strengths and vulnerabilities. The skills necessary to meet such needs are diverse and require collaborative work across disciplines and between staff from different agencies, including education, health, social services and different service providers.

Achieving much of what people with intellectual disabilities, their families, support workers and others working with people with intellectual disabilities might aspire to, in terms of social inclusion, choice and participation, will depend not just on the opportunities available to people with intellectual disabilities. Also central is ensuring, as far as is possible, sound physical and mental health, and the provision of support and communication strategies that are based on an understanding of individual need. This approach requires a clear understanding of the responsibilities of all those concerned with respect to the prevention, detection and treatment of ill health and ready access to primary and secondary health services and to specialist services as and when required. The extent of health inequalities and the attitudinal and practical barriers to primary, secondary and specialist health care services are increasingly acknowledged, if not, as yet, exactly resolved.

This book is a very welcome contribution to the literature with its specific focus on the mental health of people with intellectual disabilities. As exemplified by the different chapters, this has been an area of substantial development over the last few years. Clinicians and researchers have gained a much better recognition of the relevance of different conceptual models of understanding of the various developmental, biological, psychological and social factors that might predispose to, precipitate and/or maintain the occurrence of particular behaviours and/or abnormal mental states affecting people with intellectual disabilities, and of the range of interventions that should be considered. The focus for the early chapters is on assessment and on the complex issues that can arise with respect to consent and the capacity of individuals to consent to interventions. The subsequent chapters address various aspects of psychiatric comorbidity and focus on specific issues that are becoming increasingly relevant, particularly with respect to people with mild intellectual disabilities, such as substance misuse and the needs of those arrested, charged with and/or convicted of offences. Other chapters focus on challenging behaviour and also on the mental health needs of older people with intellectual disabilities – perhaps best exemplified by the age-related needs of people with Down's syndrome. The final chapters are on interventions and on services.

This book brings together under one cover present-day knowledge and through its very publication makes a clear statement about the importance of these issues and of what can be done. This book is fundamentally optimistic in that its emphasis is on the benefits of sound assessment and informed intervention, yet it also brings to our attention the limitations of our knowledge and the complexity of the field.

Tony Holland
April 2009

1 Introduction

Angela Hassiotis[1], Diana Andrea Barron[1] and Ian Hall[2]

[1]Department of Mental Health Services, University College London, UK
[2]East London NHS Foundation Trust, UK

Clinical involvement with, and awareness of, disability is a core component of the current undergraduate medical curriculum. It is one of eight key themes recommended by the General Medical Council which run through the entire five-year medical programme. Despite this, the majority of clinicians who only meet individuals with intellectual disabilities occasionally, often only have limited experience or training in how to work with this group where communication difficulties and variable symptom presentation create particular challenges in the consulting room.

Intellectual Disability Psychiatry: A Practical Handbook has been written and edited by working clinicians and academics in intellectual disabilities with the aim of creating a concise and practical text that addresses the clinical uncertainties that we face in everyday practice.

Working with people with intellectual disability is intellectually stimulating and professionally rewarding. All contributors have day-to-day clinical contact with people with intellectual disabilities, run diverse and innovative services and train undergraduate medical students and psychiatrists in training.

The complex clinical case work and emerging advances in epidemiological and health services research make this an exciting and interesting field. Recent government policy guidance provides an impetus for service innovation and the results of public enquiries help to prioritize initiatives to combat discrimination that people with intellectual disabilities can be subjected to when accessing health services.

People with intellectual disabilities experience high rates of mental disorders especially if problem behaviours are included in the prevalence rates. They are more likely to have associated physical health problems particularly people with more severe intellectual disabilities. There are many challenges in supporting people with intellectual disabilities overcome mental health problems. The ascertainment

Intellectual Disability Psychiatry: a practical handbook   Angela Hassiotis, Diana Andrea Barron and Ian Hall (eds)
© 2009 John Wiley & Sons, Ltd

of mental disorders in this population is far from straightforward: the existing major classification systems, ICD-10 and DSM-IV-TR, are difficult to apply because the criteria for many mental disorders assume a level of ability and development that is lacking in our population. Furthermore, onset or relapse of a mental disorder may be unrecognized because of assumptions that people with intellectual disabilities behave in a certain way. Conditions that are treatable may therefore remain untreated and consequently the individual's needs are not met and their quality of life is reduced. *Intellectual Disability Psychiatry* will enable readers to effectively challenge this diagnostic overshadowing.

Chapters cover the key topics in the psychiatry of intellectual disability and include illustrative cases and examples of good practice. Communication is the topic of our first main chapter, and returned to many times in *Intellectual Disability Psychiatry* because it is so essential. Good communication skills can make all the difference for a clinician to be able to identify mental health problems in people with intellectual disabilities, and deliver treatment interventions.

In many parts of the world, there are no specific mental health services for people with intellectual disabilities. In other places, people with intellectual disabilities use a combination of specialist and mainstream services. We hope *Intellectual Disability Psychiatry*, written from a practice perspective, will help enable all psychiatrists to have the confidence and skills to work with people with intellectual disabilities. We have designed it to be an invaluable aid in achieving professional competencies and passing professional exams such as the MRCPsych. It is also highly relevant to other health professionals and social workers working with this client group.

We have deliberately avoided making *Intellectual Disability Psychiatry* an exhaustive research guide, though references to important papers are included as well as suggestions for further reading.

Psychiatry for people with intellectual disabilities is a very well established specialty in the United Kingdom, and several of our contributors use UK legislation and services to illustrate important principles. However, the content and information presented in *Intellectual Disability Psychiatry* can be adapted and applied in other settings outside the UK. We have intentionally adopted an international perspective in our community care chapter, and solicited contributions from three continents to help ensure an outward looking, forward thinking focus.

2 Effective Communication

Diana Andrea Barron[1] and Emma Winn[2]

[1]*Department of Mental Health Sciences, University of London, UK*
[2]*Camden Learning Disabilities Service, London, UK*

2.1 Introduction

This chapter aims to give some good practice points to facilitate communication with people with intellectual disability. In reality very few practitioners will have any training specific to the communication needs of this group of people. *Our Health, Our Care, Our Say: A New Direction For Community Services* [1] drew attention to the lack of skills and training; stating that there is a need to build up skills, especially in basic communication, in social care settings where only 25% of employees have a qualification. Healthcare for All [2] recommends that training for all health care professionals at undergraduate and postgraduate level must include intellectual disabilities on the curriculum.

People communicate in a variety of different ways and all have a right to communicate. A simple definition of communication is dependent upon three things:

1. a message to communicate
2. people who need to communicate with each other
3. a shared way of communicating.

This simple definition applies to everyone regardless of their age and ability to communicate.

Understanding and improving communication can greatly enhance clinical care and the experience of people with intellectual disabilities and those working with them. Moreover recent changes in UK legislation formalize a duty upon practitioners to strive to communicate effectively with individuals in order to maximize their understanding and ability to make decisions. For this reason we hope that this chapter

Intellectual Disability Psychiatry: a practical handbook   Angela Hassiotis, Diana Andrea Barron and Ian Hall (eds)
© 2009 John Wiley & Sons, Ltd

will be used by the reader to help inform their understanding of many other parts of this textbook.

We discuss the different components of communication and the way that these impact upon the assessment and management of mental health disorders in people with intellectual disabilities. The basis of communication difficulties and their prevalence are outlined.

We also consider the general issues of communication in a clinical setting and the role of communication with others including carers, other disciplines and agencies that are frequently involved in the network working with a person with intellectual disabilities. The chapter is written from the joint perspective of psychiatry of intellectual disabilities and speech and language therapy and includes good practice points and case vignettes that can be used by readers to improve their own communication practices.

2.2 Background

There is a high incidence of communication difficulties in people with intellectual disabilities in comparison to the rest of the population. Research has indicated that anything between 50 and 90% of people with intellectual disabilities have such difficulties [3]. Therefore health professionals need to modify their communication to accommodate the communication needs of the person with intellectual disabilities. This will include spoken language, non-verbal communication such as facial expression, body language and gestures and any written forms of communication.

An approach that encompasses all the above and values all forms of communication equally is Total Communication. This is the communication approach that we have based the chapter on. The environment plays a key role in promoting effective communication. Considerations should also be made to ensure that communication is culturally appropriate with increased use of interpreters versus reliance on family members.

There is a higher incidence of sensory impairments with people with intellectual disabilities than in the general population. The literature shows that up to 60% of people with intellectual disabilities are likely to have a sensory impairment of some kind. 50% of people with intellectual disabilities were found to have a hearing impairment and between 30 and 70% have visual impairment [4, 5]. This figure can rise to 80% with certain 'at risk' groups, such as people with Down's syndrome.

There is also a higher incidence of physical disability amongst people with intellectual disabilities [2] and this can impact on communication skills. Such people are more likely to be dependent on others, therefore the ability and opportunity to communicate their needs and wishes and to have these acted upon is essential. The communication modes such as speech and signing may be more difficult for people with intellectual and physical disabilities to use easily.

From the speech and language therapist's perspective the communication skills of people with intellectual disabilities are described as:

1. **Pre-verbal:** This means that people do not have the cognitive abilities to understand words. They have profound and multiple learning disabilities. They can be helped to understand through routines, tone of voice, repetition, the context of the situation, objects and their own experience.
2. **Non-verbal:** This means that people have abilities to understand words but do not have the ability to express themselves using words and will use an alternative means, for example signing, pictures.
3. **Verbal:** People will have a variety of skills in understanding language and expressing themselves, predominantly using speech.

2.3 Professional obligations

Communication with patients, family members, carers and other professionals is an inherent part of everyday practice. There is a general assumption that both doctor and patient are able to understand what is being said and to contribute and respond in a way that is also understood. In clinical practice this assumption often does not hold true particularly in the context people with intellectual disabilities. In these situations doctors have a duty to communicate in a way that is appropriate for the individual.

This duty stems from the doctor's duty to preserve the autonomy of the patient, their right to self-determination and is a cornerstone of medical ethics. Increasingly this ethical principle has become incorporated into the law and has led to legal obligations set out in statute. See Box 2.1 for key statutes and policy applicable in England.

Box 2.1 Key statutes and policy in England

Human Rights Act 2000 [6]
Article 3: Freedom from torture or inhuman or degrading treatment
   Article 14: Freedom from discrimination

Mental Capacity Act (MCA) 2005 [7]
Principle 2: 'A person is not to be treated as unable to make a decision unless all practicable steps to help him to do so have been taken without success.' (section 1(3))

Mental Capacity Act Code of Practice 2008 [8]
The MCA Code of Practice (chapter 3) provides general guidance for communication and further guidance specific to intellectual disabilities. It emphasizes

---

the importance of doing everything practical to help a person make a decision for themselves before concluding that they lack capacity to do so. It also states that to help someone make a decision for themselves, all possible and appropriate means of communication should be tried.

Mental Health Act 2007 [9]
Section 132B(1) imposes a duty to provide 'help in obtaining information about and understanding, ... the provisions of this Act' ... and other issues relevant to the Act.

Mental Health Act 1983 Code of Practice amended 2008 [10]
Chapter 2 outlines the duty to keep patients informed of their rights. Section 2.3 in the same chapter also outlines general guidance for communication with patients and states that everything possible should be done to overcome barriers to effective communication, which may be caused.

Section 2.4 highlights how communication difficulties affect each patient individually, so that practitioners can assess the needs of each patient and address them in the most appropriate way.

Chapter 34 specifically considers the needs of people with intellectual disabilities and people with autism and highlights the need to set aside sufficient time for preparation of suitable information and for preparation before meetings. Meetings should be held in an environment that is not intimidating, in order to allow the patient every chance to understand the information given.

Valuing People 2001 [11]
In paragraph 4.30 the white paper outlines the government expectation that organizations working with people with intellectual disabilities will develop communication policies and produce and disseminate information in accessible formats. For those with severe disabilities this may require individual communication techniques and effective use of new technology.

Good Medical Practice (2006) [12]
Published by the General Medical Council, this guidance for doctors imposes the duty on doctors to make sure, wherever practical, that arrangements are made to meet patients' language and communication needs.

Seeking Consent: Working with People with Learning Disabilities (2001) [13]
Published by the Department of Health specifically looks at the issue of consent in intellectual disabilities – both those individuals with and without the capacity to make decisions for themselves.

Beyond the duty to communicate is the therapeutic importance of good communication and its role in developing a therapeutic alliance between the doctor, patient and carers and other professionals around them [14].

2.4 Language skills of people with intellectual disability

Understanding of language

Many people with intellectual disabilities will have difficulties understanding what the health professional says. Some people will have developed good social language which masks their underlying difficulties, and it is important to be aware of this. Also some people will have developed an ability to understand simple abstract questions, for example, 'What did you do today?', 'Where's so and so?', but will find it harder to understand more complex abstract questions and concepts such as inference, for example, 'What would you do if ... ?', emotions and time concepts such as 'yesterday', 'tomorrow' and 'twice a day'.

It is useful to think about understanding from a simple developmental perspective while being mindful that the health professional is working with people who are adults and who will have had many life experiences which will increase their abilities. This means that sometimes people will be able to understand at a seemingly higher level because of something that they have experienced. In Box 2.2 we outline the key stages of communication development.

Box 2.2 Stages of communication development

1. Situational – people do not understand words but may understand because of the context, someone's tone of voice, experience and because of their routine.

2. Words are guides only to things that are present, that is people do what they usually do when they hear that word or see that sign.

3. Words are still guides only, but the things that are talked about don't need to be present – they could be in the next room.

4. Familiar words are recognized and understood and linked together in a typical way. Other parts of the sentence that they do not understand are ignored.

5. Sentences are understood using rules, for example, 'order of mention'. Misunderstandings can happen. For example, 'Before you have lunch you

> need to ring your friend.' The person understands it as 'have lunch and then ring' but the friend is out when they ring.
>
> 6. Full understanding of every part of the sentence.

Often people with intellectual disabilities find it possible to understand what is being said, even though some words are not understood as they use a variety of different strategies. These include (i) their familiarity with the context or person speaking, (ii) guessing, (iii) understanding the speaker's non-verbal cues such as body language, facial expression and gestures or signing.

Box 2.3　Learning point

Think about what it is like when you are in a country where you understand only a little of the language. What helps you?

1. People talking slowly and giving you time to process what is being said.

2. People using everyday vocabulary, short sentences and simple grammar.

3. Non-verbal signals such as tone of voice, gesture or miming.

4. People using objects and pictures to explain.

5. The context of the situation, that is time of day, place.

Spoken language

People's ability to express themselves and the way in which they do it will vary. People may have difficulties in putting sentences together, a reduced vocabulary or unclear speech. This will mean that people with intellectual disabilities may have difficulties making themselves understood and the health professional may have difficulties understanding what the person is saying particularly if they do not know each other.

Due to neurological differences, some people with intellectual disabilities will have difficulties with pronunciation. People with physical disabilities such as cerebral palsy may have dysarthric speech. This means that the person has weakness in the speech musculature and difficulties with breath support for talking. Their speech maybe characterized by imprecise articulation or mis-articulation. Other groups such as people with Down's syndrome may have articulation difficulties due to their anatomical differences such as high arched palate and low tongue muscle tone. Other causes of speech difficulties beyond the scope of this chapter include immature speech processes (phonology), dyspraxia and dysfluency.

Non-verbal communication

Non-verbal communication is very powerful and people gain much information from the non-verbal part of the message. Argyle and Alkema [15] found that verbal language provided 7% of the information whereas body language provided 55% and tone, pitch and intonation 38%. Types of non-verbal communication include body language, facial expression, gestures, signing, behaviour, tone, pitch and intonation. Arguably it is these methods of communication that are most difficult to interpret. During clinical practice they are largely dependent on the professional's familiarity with the person with whom they are working, which is often limited. An example where these non-verbal forms of communication have been used in conjunction with joint working with carers and support workers who know the client well is the Disability Distress Assessment Tool (DisDAT) [16] (Box 2.4).

Box 2.4   Good practice example – the Disability Distress Assessment Tool

A palliative care team working with people with intellectual disabilities developed the Disability Distress Assessment Tool (DisDAT). The tool enables clinicians to record the number and severity of distress behaviours and provides a check list to facilitate the process of identifying and treating possible causes of distress. Distress behaviours include vocalizations, speech, habits, posture and body observations including: pulse, respiratory rate, appetite and sleep. It was initially devised for people with intellectual disabilities requiring input from palliative care. It has been used in the assessment and management of other groups.

The health professional's non-verbal communication skills are particularly important when working with people with intellectual disabilities who do not always understand everything that is said. For example, if you are talking about something serious then your facial expression should be similarly serious otherwise there is a danger that the person will misinterpret what you are saying. The health professional's body language is a tool that can be used to enhance communication with a person with intellectual disability. It can be used to be encouraging, for example, open body posture, sitting down at the person's level, particularly if they are in a wheelchair, to maintain appropriate eye contact.

The following case vignettes are used to illustrate common non-verbal communication in clinical practice.

Case vignette 2.1

A man called Fred who is non-verbal and can understand some single words but mostly understands through watching people and the context. He had been offered a drink with no sugar. The worker took sugar so she went and got it for herself. Fred saw this and held out his cup to indicate he wanted sugar too.

Fred is aware of the environment that he is in and notices the worker's behaviour. He uses a gesture to get sugar as a substitute for the words, 'Can I have some sugar'.

Case vignette 2.2

A woman called Sally who has some single words and short phrases was interacting with a worker who got up and put her coat on. Sally said, 'Bye' and pushed the worker to the door. Sally could not say, 'I'll show you out' so physically did so.

In this scenario Sally will have noticed the worker's body language as the worker stood up to leave; Sally used behaviour to substitute for the phrase 'I'll show you out'. This scenario also illustrates the potential for behaviours to be misinterpreted as challenging behaviour rather than a means of communication.

Box 2.5   Maximizing communication for people who are pre-verbal or who have limited understanding

1. Regular routines/timetables that people can anticipate.

2. Repetition of an activity so that people can start to predict what is going to happen and join in.

3. Tone of voice will help people to understand whether something is serious or funny.

4. Facial expression – make sure the expression matches what is being said.

5. Familiar situations and familiar rooms/buildings/places.

6. Sensory cues including sounds, smells and visuals cues.

7. Objects of reference – these are often real objects that symbolize something that regularly happens to help the person understand what is going to happen, for example, a person who goes swimming every week is shown their swimming trunks before they leave the house.

Use of language/social interaction

Some people with intellectual disabilities have more difficulties with using language in an appropriate manner, particularly people with autism. They may use learnt phrases or echo what is being said or echo something that they have heard from their past experience (delayed echolalia). In the clinical setting it is the responsibility of the health professional to ascertain how the person likes to be communicated with.

Written language

Although literacy skills are often reduced in this client group many people can understand written information if they have support, especially if it is written in an accessible way with pictures, symbols and photos. Using the 'Top Tips' in Box 2.6 will help make written information easier to read.

Box 2.6   Top tips for written information

1. Information should be relevant. Cut out anything that is not needed or is confusing.

2. Keep your sentences short. Use one clause per sentence. Try not to use conjunctions such as: but, therefore, because. Use 'and' only if you are writing a short list: eggs, milk and cheese. For longer lists, use bullet points.

3. Use plain English. Avoid jargon, technical language, abbreviations (apart from very common ones, e.g. TV, BBC) or difficult words. A long word can often be replaced with a short one, for example 'hard' not 'difficult', 'use' not 'utilize'.

4. Be consistent. Use the same words and phrases even if this seems repetitive. Use words and phrases that this client group will be familiar with.

5. If the person needs to do something, show this clearly. Use bold text or a bullet point.

6. Use numbers, for example '5', rather than words.

7. Lay the text out clearly, with plenty of white space.

8. Use Arial typeface and larger print – 16 point.

9. Do not use block capitals or italics or underlining as they are more difficult to read. Highlight important words in bold.

2.5 The impact of context on communication

Context refers to the physical environment or the emotional environment of the individuals. The physical environment can easily be manipulated in most circumstances. Ideally this would be quiet and comfortable. In the context of derilium, medical students are taught to interview the patient in a quiet brightly lit environment, thereby minimizing potential sources of distraction and opportunities for misinterpreting visual stimuli. The rationale for this approach is that the acutely confused patient has difficulty concentrating and maintaining selective attention. In specific disorders such as autism there is impairment of the attentional and perceptual abilities of the individual. This may present as an inability to focus on one thing or difficulty attending to additional extraneous stimuli such as the sound of advancing traffic when crossing the road. Many individuals including those with autism have sensory hypersensitivities (hyperacusis); these may be to touch, smell, sound and visual stimuli. This may cause distress to the individual and may be the origin of some challenging behaviours.

It is also important to consider the emotional environment for the individual. Emotional regulation can be challenging for many individuals. In states of emotional arousal such as anxiety secondary to pain or an unfamiliar environment, it can be difficult to participate in any exchange of communication in a meaningful way that enables the individual to both understand and remember what was said. In order to improve communication in these scenarios, individuals are usually able to regulate their own emotions. This requires the individual to be able recognize their internal state, to communicate that state and to be able to regulate their own response to it.

Studies show that strategies to regulate emotion are present from as early as infancy where rudimentary strategies such as looking away from aversive stimuli are used. For individuals with intellectual disabilities emotional self-regulation is largely dependent on the individual's cognitive abilities, social skills and previous experiences. It can be useful to adopt a developmental perspective when considering an individual's emotional environment and its likely impact on any interview or assessment.

Case vignette 2.3

David has moderate intellectual disability and autism; he is seen by the community psychiatrist in the health promotion room and spends the duration of the meeting rearranging leaflets. He is therefore not able to attend to the questions that he has been asked.

In this scenario David has difficulty maintaining selective attention; because he is anxious or because he has autism and because there are too many competing stimuli in the environment for him to attend to. As a result of this it is likely that David will not communicate as effectively as he is able to.

The detail of how to apply communication skills to the psychiatric consultation with people with intellectual disabilities is covered in Chapter 3. However Box 2.7 gives some essential pointers.

Box 2.7   What will help health professionals to understand?

1. Ask the person if they have any communication aids, for example, a communication passport which describes how they communicate

2. Make sure you are listening carefully.

3. Make sure you are looking at the person when they are talking.

4. If you cannot understand, try to make the person feel at ease by saying, 'Sometimes it is difficult for me to understand. Could you say it again, please.'

5. Don't pretend to understand when you have not.

6. Ask the person if it is OK to ask the carer/support worker for help with communication.

7. As you get to know the person you will find it easier to understand them.

2.6 Working with others

Working with others is a central feature of modern medical practice. The role of the collateral history in the assessment, examination and management of patients is an important skill in all medical disciplines. Increasingly doctors work within multidisciplinary and multi-agency teams which can facilitate the communication between different disciplines in the care of their client group. In the field of intellectual disabilities this should be no different. However in the context of more severe intellectual disabilities, the clinician becomes more reliant on the information provided by others.

The collateral history enables the clinician to gather a longitudinal history. Consulting with carers will provide in-depth knowledge including the person's likes/dislikes, distress signs and signals, allergies, work, social history and medical history. Further to this carers and others may be involved in monitoring the progress of the person and will therefore require information and understanding of the assessment/treatment in order to be able to support the patient to make use of any intervention and to maximize the efficacy of an assessment/treatment. The recognition of the carer's role has grown in importance as reflected by legislation. For example the Mental Capacity Act (MCA) 2005 in England and Wales requires the involvement of carers in the process of making best interest decisions for those who lack mental capacity. *Carers at the Heart of 21st-Century Families and Communities* [17] extends the rights of carers, and professionals' obligations towards them.

When consulted, carers have expressed their frustration with the way that professionals communicate with them [18]. Most frequently criticized is the information given to them, and repetition of questions asked by professionals. Various approaches have been implemented to reduce repetition and improve the effectiveness of information exchange and communication for patients, professionals and services. Here four approaches adopted in services in the UK – Health Action Plans, Person Centred Planning, the Single Assessment Process and the Care Programme Approach (CPA) – are described.

The Health Action Plan is a patient-held document that has been devised with the patient in a format that is accessible and meaningful for them and explains any actions needed to maintain and improve their health. It is described as a mechanism to link the individual and the range of services and supports they need, in order to get better health. Health Action Plans were introduced in England following the white paper *Valuing People* which proposed that all people with intellectual disabilities would have a Health Action Plan by the year 2005 [19].

Valuing People also proposed that Person Centred Planning should become a central process in intellectual disabilities services. It is an approach to ensure that services provide support in the way the person wants and puts them at the centre of the process. It helps people plan for the future and enables people to become more involved in their communities. Person Centred Planning encourages effective communication with individuals that enables individuals to express their needs, preferences and ambitions in a way that is understandable to them and others in their network of professional support and friends. Services are developing individual approaches to Person Centred Planning. One approach is to use Person Centred Thinking tools [20] which include:

• what's working/what's not working

• what's important to the person and for the person

• hopes and dreams

• communication charts

• relationship circle

These tools, plus a variety of others, help an organization build up practices that encourage its employees to listen to the person and to find out what they want.

The Single Assessment Process aims to support person centred assessment and management of care for adults who have health and social care needs. It was introduced to the care of older people in 2001 following the national framework for care of older people and subsequently has been adopted by other services including community learning disability teams and forensic services. The Single Assessment Process comprises the following components:

• a single point of entry to the service

• a holistic assessment of needs including health, social care and carers' needs

• care planning

• delivery of care

• and subsequent review

The Single Assessment Process provides a framework that can coordinate the assessment of the health and social care needs of an individual and supports the communication and sharing of information between health and social care agencies.

The Care Programme Approach (CPA) is a co-ordinated approach to care planning that is provided for all individuals who have severe and enduring mental health needs. This is adapted for use in intellectual disabilities services for people with severe mental health needs in addition to their intellectual disabilities. Box 2.8 describes an example of this where a service improved the CPA process to make it more accessible and person centred. All materials were devised and piloted with people with intellectual disabilities, and each topic of discussion uses accessible language and has an accompanying picture which matches the CPA headings [21, 22].

Box 2.8 Good practice example – the four stages of the CLDS CPA toolkit [16]

- Stage 1: The CPA co-ordinator meets the person at least two weeks before the CPA meeting to talk through the outcomes of their last meeting and to plan what the person would like to talk about at the next CPA meeting, using the accessible agenda and photos of professionals involved in the person's care to talk about who will be there. The 'What is a CPA?' leaflet can be used to support the person to explain what the meeting is about.

- Stage 2: The person leads their CPA meeting using the planned accessible agenda to introduce each topic. The discussion is structured using 'what's working/not working' flip charts and it is completed during the meeting by the person with support as required or the care coordinator.

- Stage 3: The CPA co-ordinator transfers all handwritten data onto an accessible CPA form for the person and the local NHS trust CPA form for professionals.

- Stage 4: The CPA co-ordinator meets with the person to talk through the meeting and the outcomes using the signed and completed accessible CPA form. This is their record of the meeting and a copy is left with the person.

2.7 Conclusion

Communication is an intrinsic part of any clinical interaction. This chapter has provided an overview of communication development and difficulties and aims to provide the health professional with a range of resources to be used in their clinical setting. Box 2.9 summarizes the key points for communicating effectively with people with intellectual disabilities.

Box 2.9 Top tips for communication

1. Speak slowly; using everyday words, simple grammar and short sentences, that is plain English with no jargon.

---

2. Use pictures/photographs to help explain or draw pictures.

3. Link your explanation with everyday things especially if you need to talk about more abstract things such as time concepts. For example, 'take your tablet three times a day' is more easily understood as 'take your tablets at breakfast, lunch and dinner.'

4. Write the key information down and then people can go through it with a friend/carer/support worker afterwards.

5. Be aware of your facial expression and body language. Are they giving the same message as your speech? Use lots of non-verbal feedback, especially head nods and facial expression to show that you're listening.

6. People with intellectual disabilities may have difficulty ignoring distractions. Make sure you are talking to them in a quiet place.

7. Think about how to ask questions. Remember that open questions can be more difficult. Closed questions, that is yes/no questions, are often not helpful as people may answer 'yes' because they think you want them to say yes. Either/or questions may be easier, but keep them short, so that they don't just repeat the last thing you said, for example, 'Do you like tea or orange juice?'

8. Give the person plenty of time to respond; you might have to wait longer than you'd expect.

9. Check that they have understood you. You may need to ask them to repeat back what you said. Some people will find this hard to do.

10. Be aware of other things that may affect communication, for example hearing, vision, physical and mental health, epilepsy, medication, time of day (are they a 'morning' person?) general mood, interest in the topic.

11. Be sensitive to any cultural 'rules' the person may have, particularly with regard to eye contact, personal space and gestures that may have different meanings. Check what language the person is most familiar with and whether you need an interpreter.

Acknowledgements

Richard Lohan, accessible information worker, Camden Learning Disability Service.
    Sue Martin, highly specialist speech and language therapist, Camden Learning Disabilities Service.

References

1. Department of Health (2006) *Our Health, Our Care, Our Say: A New Direction for Community Services*, The Stationery Office, London, p. 188.
2. Michael, J. (chair) (2008) Healthcare for All: Report of the Independent Enquiry into Access to Health Care for People with Learning Disabilities, Available at www.iahpld.org.uk (last accessed 28 January 2009) pp. 34–36.
3. Bhaumik, S., Watson, J.M., Thorp, C.F. *et al.* (2008) Body Mass Index in adults with intellectual disability: distribution, associations and service implications: a population based prevalence study. *Journal of Intellectual Disability Research*, **52** (4), 287–298.
4. Carvill, S. (2001) Sensory impairments, intellectual disability and psychiatry. *Journal of Intellectual Disability Research*, **45** (6), 467–483.
5. Owens, P.L., Kerker, B.D., Zigler, E. and Horwtiz, S.M. (2006) Vision and oral health needs of individuals with intellectual disability. *Mental Retardation and Developmental Research Reviews*, **12**, 28–40.
6. Great Britain (1998) *Human Rights Act*, The Stationery Office, London.
7. Great Britain *Mental Capacity Act 2005*, The Stationery Office, London.
8. Department for Constitutional Affairs Health (2007) *Mental Capacity Act (2005) Code of Practice 2008*, London, The Stationery Office.
9. Great Britain *Mental Health Act 1986 (amended 2007)*, The Stationery Office, London.
10. Department of Health (2008) *Mental Health Act 1983 Code of Practice amended 2008*, The Stationery Office, London.
11. Department of Health (2001) *Valuing People 2001*, The Stationery Office, London.
12. General Medical Council (2006) Good Medical Practice, available on line at http://www.gmc-uk.org/guidance/good_medical_practice/index.asp.
13. Department of Health (2001) *Seeking Consent: Working with People with Learning Disabilities*, The Stationery Office, London.
14. Waitzkin, H. (1984) Doctor-patient communication: clinical implications of social scientific research. *Journal of the American Medical Association*, **252**, 2441–2446.
15. Argyle, M. and Alkema, F. (1971) The communication of friendly and hostile attitudes by verbal and non verbal signals. *European Journal of Psychology*, **1** (3), 385–402.
16. Regnard, C., Reynolds, J., Watson, B. *et al.* (2007) Understanding distress in people with severe communication difficulties: developing and assessing the Disability Distress Assessment Tool (DisDAT). *Journal of Intellectual Disability Research*, **51** (4), 277–292.
17. Department of Health (2008) *Carers at the Heart of 21st Century Families and Communities: A Caring System on Your Side, A Life of Your Own*, The Stationery Office, London.
18. Michael, J. (chair) (2008) Healthcare for All: Report of the Independent Enquiry into Access to Health Care for People with Learning Disabilities, available from hptt://www.iahpld.org.uk, pp. 17–19.

19. Department of Health (2002) *Action for Health – Health Action Plans and Health Facilitation Detailed Good Practice Guidance on Implementation for Intellectual Disability Partnership Boards*, The Stationery Office, London.

20. Sanderson, H., Smull, M. and Harvey, J. (2008) Person centred thinking, in *Person Centred Practice for Professionals* (eds J. Thompson, J. Kilbane and H. Sanderson), Open University Press, Maidenhead, pp. 45–73.

21. Department of Health (1996) *An Audit Pack for Monitoring the Care Programme Approach*, The Stationery Office, London.

22. Hall, I., Burns, E., Martin, S. *et al.* (2009) Making care programme approach meetings more accessible and person-centred for people with learning disabilities. *Advances in Mental Health and Learning Disabilities*, **3** (1), 22–28.

Further reading

Thompson, J., Kilbane, J. and Sanderson, H. (eds) *Person Centred Practice for Professionals*, Open University Press, Maidenhead.

Healthcare for All: Report of the Independent Enquiry into Access to Health Care for People with Learning Disabilities, available at www.iahpld.org.uk.

Department for constitutional affairs (2007) *Mental Capacity Act (2005) Code of Practice 2008*, The Stationery Office, London.

3 Clinical Assessment

Neill Simpson

East Dunbartonshire JLDT, UK

3.1 Introduction

A valid history is fundamental for clinical assessment. The aim of this chapter is to offer a systematic approach to assist health professionals in assessing mental disorders in adults with intellectual disability. To obtain an accurate history about a person with intellectual disability requires the collation of information from multiple sources, and sometimes the reconciliation of discordant information. Therefore, self-report should be supplemented with the observations and interpretations of informants and previous records about previous episodes of illness, treatment and outcome. Examination of the mental state is also essential, and investigation using standardized assessment tools is also useful if the tools have been validated for the purpose and are used correctly. Good communication is an essential skill in clinical assessment, and this chapter assumes knowledge of the preceding Chapter 2 about communication.

3.2 Preparing for the assessment

Even the most experienced clinician requires more time to assess a person with intellectual disability than a person of normal intellectual development. Interviews should be scheduled to be long enough to establish good communication, but not so long as to fatigue the patient, so several interviews may be needed to complete the assessment.

Information gathering

Obtain, read and summarize all the records that you can find relating to the person's development and health, and any risks there may be. Records should be obtained

Intellectual Disability Psychiatry: a practical handbook Angela Hassiotis, Diana Andrea Barron and Ian Hall (eds)
© 2009 John Wiley & Sons, Ltd

Table 3.1 Developmental milestones

Typical developmental milestones in children without developmental disabilities	6 months	12 months	24 months
Posture and large movements	Pulls to sit with no head lag	Walks to the side holding furniture	Kicks ball forward
Vision and fine movements	Watches adult move, reaches for toy	Grasps with thumb and finger	Scribbles spontaneously
Hearing and language	Vocalizes with two syllables	Imitates speech sounds	Points to one named body part
Social behaviour and play	Smiles spontaneously	Initially shy with strangers	Copies domestic activities with simultaneous play. Uses spoon, spilling little

from hospitals, schools and any other source where there has been an objective assessment of the person's abilities, health and social functioning. Try to obtain contemporaneous evidence about the person's developmental milestones (Table 3.1) and about their best stable level of functioning in adulthood, which represents their developmental level. Most people with severe or profound intellectual impairment have continuous contact with professional services from childhood onwards, and records should exist. General practitioners often have files containing paediatric and child health records.

Interview setting

Choose the most appropriate setting for the interview. Everyone communicates most effectively in a familiar environment because it reduces anxiety associated with uncertainty: it makes the fewest demands on cognitive function, and environmental cues can be referred to by gesture. Initial assessments are usually most successful in an environment that is familiar to the person with intellectual disability, such as their home or at a day service they use. Do not assume that it is safe for a clinician to visit an unfamiliar person in an environment that is unfamiliar to the clinician: you must be part of a team that has procedures to promote safe practice (usually described in a lone-worker policy). Emergencies may have to be assessed in a setting where safety can be assured, such as an emergency department of a hospital. If a patient needs continuing psychiatric treatment and review, it is often possible to use a clinic once the person is accustomed to communicating with you.

Giving information

You should provide information to referrers, and to the patient and to people providing their support, to explain what the purpose of the meeting is, and what information you will require. Much of this is applicable to every referral, so leaflets may be useful for referrers and for carers and for patients who can use written information. Some clinicians include a photograph printed on the appointment letter with the intention of improving accessibility.

3.3 Establishing communication

When eliciting a history from a person with an intellectual disability, remember that many people with significant intellectual impairment will not consistently be able to use conventional time concepts, and explicit time anchors to actual events will need to be used (see below). Past experiences, life events, additional disabilities and the environment in which the person lives all impact on their ability to communicate their distress and emotional states. Disability associated with impairment of intellectual development may also be confused with other disabilities that affect communication.

Case vignette 3.1

Charles was 60 when he was referred for assessment of declining memory. He had been deaf all of his life (prelingual deafness) and communication was through a support worker who understood his limited vocabulary of signs. Assessment earlier in his life had been inadequate, so that his intellectual ability was not known. He had been sent to an institution in childhood where education did not include sign language. He had learnt most of the skills required for activities of daily living and had been able to manage his own financial affairs. Inaccurate assessment of his abilities in the past had resulted in inappropriate services that failed to promote his development, and made assessment of declining function very difficult because comparison information was lacking.

Communication styles

Communication styles of interviewees

Communication styles that often interfere with communication are acquiescence, suggestibility, denial, fabrication, digression and disengagement (Table 3.2). The

Table 3.2 Communication styles

Acquiescence	Giving an affirmative answer to every question
Suggestibility	Guessing the reply that is expected by the interviewer
Denial	Avoidance of describing an undesired situation
Fabrication	Describing a state which differs from reality
Digression	Changing the subject, but continuing to communicate on another topic
Disengagement	Not taking part in the process of communication (in someone who is otherwise known to have the ability to communicate)

function of giving a response is not just to provide information; it includes, for example acknowledging that interaction is occurring, maintaining self-respect and the respect of others, responding to a desire to please the interviewer, avoiding unwanted consequences, concealing an undesired state (such as disability or lack of knowledge) and seeking to avoid unpleasant emotions. There is an overlap between the response styles listed; and more than one may occur within the same interview.

If a person has no spoken language it is important to enquire how they show different forms of distress including pain, nausea, fear and sadness. Ask if the person indicates location by pointing, rubbing or hitting the place. Ask specifically about toothache and headache – these are such frequent causes of pain in everybody that carers ought to be able to report them if they know the person well and the person is capable of distinguishing these symptoms. If it is impossible to distinguish these symptoms, then identifying the source of distress requires a systematic search through a list of likely causes.

If the person is able to distinguish but not describe different forms of bodily discomfort, use non-verbal methods such as gesture ('show me', 'put your hand where it is sore'). Pictures or models to show the part of the body require the person to be able to map their own body onto the representation, which requires more skill. If the person has a hearing aid, make sure they are wearing it and have it switched on. If they are accustomed to using a communication aid such as a 'talker' (speech synthesizer) it may be possible to undertake a clinical interview with a person whose speech is not understandable. Other aids to communication may be relevant, such as the use of objects of reference, communication passports and health passports.

Communication styles of informants

Do not assume that information is more accurate because it is provided by an articulate and fluent witness. Conspicuous abnormalities are more likely to be reported than subtle ones, especially if they are socially intrusive or undesired. Some features may be non-specific such as restlessness or sleep disturbance, and associated distress may be overlooked, leading to an imprecise diagnosis such as 'agitation' or 'behavioural problem'. A more precise diagnosis such as depressive disorder may be missed, if the clinician does not elicit from the informant more specific symptoms such as suicidal thoughts.

Communication styles of doctors

Diagnostic classifications in psychiatry emphasize information obtained from self-report. This can encourage doctors to disregard the non-verbal features of illness in people with intellectual disabilities. Diagnostic features that distinguish one disorder from another may not be salient to the patient. A patient with hallucinations may be troubled most by fear and sleep disturbance, and wonder why doctors repeatedly ask questions about whether the voices speak in second or third person: the patient may feel that the doctor is not paying attention to their concerns.

Discordant information

Multiple sources of information are likely to have some areas of disagreement. For example a carer may confidently assert that there are no sleep problems, which is contradicted by another carer. Such disagreements may be reconciled by collating multiple sources of information, which should be recorded and explored further by seeking dates and duration of specific examples. The health professional may discover a fluctuating condition, rather than contradictory information.

3.4 Starting the assessment

Respectful attention

Identify yourself and show your intellectual disabilities when you first meet. Explain who has requested the referral and explain the purpose of meeting. Explain, at the outset, both to the individual with intellectual disability and their carer(s) how much time you have available.

Establish eye contact, give a social greeting and offer to shake hands. The offer may not be accepted for several reasons; a person with autism or with profound intellectual impairment may not understand the meaning of the gesture, and a person who is suspicious or hostile may wish to show that they do not trust you yet. People sometimes inappropriately describe a visit by a clinician in terms that amount to a threat and you may find out later what is the reason for this. A handshake makes an important contribution to the examination of mental state, so consider offering to shake hands at the end of the interview, too, but if the gesture is not accepted, do not persevere to cause embarrassment.

Address the patient by name, using their title (Mr, Miss, etc.), until you find out if they prefer another form of address. Speak to the person who has been referred first, before speaking to other people who are present, even if the other people ask to speak to you in private. They should speak in front of the person, or they should wait until after you have spent some time with the person. The only exception should be if there is a risk that someone would come to harm by doing differently, and if that is the case consider withdrawing to prepare for the interview in a different way. Consider offering to see the person on their own for at least part of the interview. Ask for the person's consent to speak to other people about them, and if they refuse consent you should respect their refusal unless the situation falls within an area in professional guidance (e.g. from the General Medical Council) that permits or requires you to override lack of consent.

Other courtesies to be observed include explaining about writing notes during the interview, and explaining the possibility of receiving an emergency call on your mobile phone, which should be switched on (for your own safety). Try to schedule your interviews to minimize interruptions.

Introductory questions

To demonstrate that the interviewer is taking an interest in the person, ask the person about activities they enjoy, including physical activities, social activities and activities that the person gives attention to. This provides a few minutes of conversation to enable you to assess the person's language skills and engagement with the interview and to complete a mental state examination.

Make a statement of transition (Table 3.3) and explain that you want to find out about their health. If the question 'How are you?' receives a social response such as 'Very well, thank you', acknowledge it. Next ask about how the person is feeling on the day of the interview, and acknowledge and note each symptom that is described. You need to obtain both a full list of symptoms and sufficient detail about each, and be flexible about the sequence in which you do those tasks. If the patient is willing to follow your direction, it is better to obtain the full list of symptoms before detailing each.

Question sequence

Organize the sequence of questions in a way that flows naturally from common non-specific symptoms to ones that are more difficult to describe [1]. If a symptom is mentioned that does not follow this sequence, follow the patient. If symptoms are described that are irrelevant to your assessment, simply acknowledge them and write a list, without inviting more detail. When symptoms are given that are relevant to

Table 3.3 How to make a transition

Process	Explanation
Recapitulate	Repeat the main pieces of information
Check	Is the information accurate and complete?
Summarize	Give a sentence explaining your understanding of the information
Check	Ask the patient what they understood of your summary
Make a transitional statement	Explain the change of focus. 'Now I want to talk about …'

your assessment, acknowledge each one that emerges, make a note of it and invite more detail ('Tell me more about that').

Commence with questions that do not require psychological introspection. Invite the person to describe bodily symptoms followed by functions such as sleeping and eating. Next ask about common non-specific symptoms of psychological dysfunction, such as tiredness, irritability and poor concentration. Then focus on the most common symptoms of emotional disturbance, including worries (about health, family, relationships, money, work, etc.). Ask about anxiety symptoms including tension and panic. Next ask about symptoms of depression including low mood, loss of confidence, low self-esteem, hopelessness and thoughts of self-harm.

Next ask about the rare but important symptoms of mental ill health if they have not been previously mentioned: problems with memory, abnormal experiences such as seeing or hearing things that other people don't, feeling that someone is against you or trying to harm you, feeling forced to do something you don't want to.

Time anchors

It requires more cognitive effort to reconstruct the history in sequence than to list the symptoms according to the degree of concern they cause the patient at the present time, and this cognitive effort should be made by the doctor, not the patient. You can obtain the sequence by identifying a time when the person was well or by choosing an 'anchor event' that allows the person and informants to recall what the person was doing and feeling on a particular date. Public holidays, birthdays and other non-routine events or visits are useful examples to offer to create anchors. You can then construct a history forward in time from the anchor.

Questioning style

Be aware that the questioning words (what, which, who, where, when, how, why) are not equally easy to answer – the sequence listed here represents the usual order of difficulty. If possible, frame your questions to avoid the more difficult forms, and sequence your interview to get information using descriptions of what the person was doing and feeling before asking anything about when or why. Obtain information using open questions and prompts ('Tell me what you feel') before asking closed questions ('Were you crying?') and try to ask for only one piece of information per question. If you ask the person to choose a response ('Are you happy or sad?'), there is a greater chance of them choosing the second response than the first, so you might get a different answer if you give the choice in the opposite sequence. And do not be surprised if the acquiescent response to that question is 'yes'.

Be alert for problems due to response styles. Abandon a topic that is causing disruption to the flow of conversation, and do not try to persevere with a standard checklist of symptoms if the person's attention is elsewhere; the replies will be invalid. Try following the topic that the interviewee wishes to discuss to see if it reveals more symptoms; or resume a discussion about 'what you like doing' to re-engage the person's attention in the conversation.

Try to ensure that each interview finishes with the interviewee feeling it was a positive experience that they are willing to do again. Sometimes, if the interview is difficult, decide not to finish the task during one session, and instead focus on re-establishing a positive relationship to enable assessment to continue another time.

3.5 Presenting problems

Mental health problems usually present with symptoms. A symptom is an experience which is a change from the person's usual state, out of keeping with the situation, associated with distress or disability, which does not cease at will [2]. For people with intellectual disabilities it is not always possible to ascertain the extent of voluntary control. Specialists in this field consider it sufficient to identify a symptom if there is a description by the person of an unwelcome change [3].

When a patient with intellectual disability consults a doctor, a communication problem may arise if the doctor focuses on the developmental problem and ignores a newly acquired problem, whereas the patient is likely to wish to focus on the new problem. Overlooking diagnosable conditions because the doctor focuses on a developmental disorder is called 'diagnostic overshadowing'.

Case vignette 3.2

A community learning disability nurse was asked to give advice about Harold, a middle-aged man with severe intellectual disability who had a lifelong problem of being distractible and impulsive. The patient had recently become agitated, and had developed facial flushing. The nurse advised carers to make an appointment with the GP to ask if he might have a physical health problem. The GP prescribed an antipsychotic drug and referred the patient to a psychiatrist to assess 'problem behaviour'.

In addition to diagnostic overshadowing, case vignette 3.2 also illustrates 'baseline exaggeration', meaning that the evidence that a person has become unwell is an exacerbation of a pre-existing problem. Therefore, it is imperative to gather information about the presenting problem as well as about the person's development and thus compare the person's current functioning with their best developmental level in order to make an accurate diagnosis.

Case vignette 3.3

David, a young man with mild intellectual disability, was interviewed as part of a research project. The interview enquired only about problems observed in the past month. The person described rapid thoughts and speech and other symptoms meeting the research criteria for mania, if they represented change. When the interviewer asked the person's mother about the symptoms, she confirmed them and added that he had always had problems of impulsivity, distractibility and poor emotional control, and she believed that her son had undiagnosed attention deficit hyperactivity disorder (ADHD).

The features of developmental disorders overlap with the features of acquired disorders. This can cause errors unless you complete the diagnosis of the developmental disorder first. No matter the order in which you obtain the information, ensure that you have obtained enough information to assess both developmental and acquired disorders before you reach a conclusion about diagnoses, bearing in mind that developmental disorders do not protect a person from acquiring additional disorders – quite the reverse.

Case vignette 3.4

Parveen is a young woman who was referred from adolescent mental health services with a diagnosis of autism in the context of mild intellectual disabilities. She was described as having problems of emotional and behavioural disturbance related to autism and had been prescribed an antipsychotic drug. After a series of crises (including assaulting her mother and sister, setting fire to her mother's clothing in the kitchen and running away) she was admitted to hospital. It was decided to reduce the dose of medication, and within a few weeks she started expressing bizarre beliefs and responding to auditory hallucinations. A review of her developmental history revealed that the features of abnormal communication and reciprocal social interaction had not been observed before adolescence. A diagnosis of schizophrenia had not been made in adolescence, perhaps because English was not the first language of her family, and some of her beliefs were assumed to be culturally determined. She had been given medication that suppressed symptoms before any diagnosis had been made.

To the extent to which the person can describe symptoms, apply the approach used with other people of the same age. For each symptom find out the frequency and duration, onset, maximum intensity, changes in intensity over time and associations between symptoms. Do not assume that anyone can attribute the cause of their symptoms precisely; explore the range of possible causes, including life events and stresses, physical illness and adverse effects of medication.

Situations where symptoms are described insufficient to make a diagnosis

The most frequently described symptoms of mental ill health are non-specific. There may be a clear change in the person's well-being, but too few features to make a diagnosis with a standard classification such as ICD-10 or DSM-IV. The most satisfactory solution is to use a modified system such as DC-LD [3]. If there are insufficient symptoms for DC-LD but the patient clearly has a change of mental functioning associated with distress or disability, make a provisional diagnosis using non-verbal phenomena of illness to allow one to choose effective treatment.

Problem behaviour

Referrals for psychiatric assessment are often framed in terms of behavioural problems, rather than symptoms or signs. There is a great deal of jargon about this subject. Try to maintain an open mind about the possible role of ill health. Do not accede to other people's assumption that every problem behaviour is a disorder (with the expectation that there is medication that will stop the behaviour); do not be distracted by premature explanations of the function of behaviour such as 'demand-avoidance' or 'attention-seeking'; and do not dismiss anything as 'just behavioural'.

A behavioural history requires an objective description of what the person actually does (do not write 'aggressive behaviour', if the description is 'he hits with his clenched fist without aiming'). The form of the behaviour should be described as precisely as possible, which generally means describing the consequences. Each item of behaviour should be listed together with the frequency, duration and intensity. This is not as objective as early behavioural psychologists hoped: if a person throws a cup close to another person and it smashes on the wall, should it be described as violence with the use of an inaccurately aimed missile, or destructive behaviour reckless of the safety of others, or a carefully executed attempt at intimidation? Working out the function of the behaviour is often conjectural, and unfortunately there is no satisfactory taxonomy of functions.

Enquire about behaviour that harms others including assaultative behaviour; behaviour that harms the person themselves (usually called self-injurious behaviour); behaviour that causes damage to the environment (destructive behaviour); socially disruptive behaviour (including noise, absconding, interfering with other people's property, faecal smearing); abnormal eating (such as pica); and repetitive non-functional behaviour (such as tics and stereotypies). Enquire about behaviour harmful to health (smoking tobacco, using excessive alcohol, using non-prescribed drugs) and offending behaviour (such as theft, inappropriate sexual behaviour and fire-setting).

The detailed assessment of behaviour problems, including functional behavioural analysis, is described in Chapter 9.

Intermittent problems

Transient symptoms are common. Migraine and asthma are likely to be as frequent among people with intellectual disabilities as in the rest of the population. Anxiety disorders including panic may be more prevalent, and epilepsy definitely so. Adequate assessment of paroxysmal disorders requires the person providing the information to record the sequence of features from the first manifestations until recovery. For epilepsy it is essential that information is obtained from a person who has directly witnessed a seizure. If the information is not available at the time of the interview, provide a written list of the information you require, or perhaps arrange to speak on the phone to a person who has the information.

3.6 Background history

Most people receiving specialist intellectual disability services will have had an assessment by a school and by a member of a multidisciplinary team. This should include much of the relevant background, and a description of support needs and risks.

If the assessment has not previously been done, or information is missing, it needs to be gathered, perhaps with the support of the community intellectual disability team.

Medical history

Some disorders that are infrequent in the general population are more prevalent among people with intellectual disabilities, and may be related to the cause of the disability. For example, thyroid disease is common among people with Down's syndrome at all ages, and epilepsy is associated with several disorders that cause developmental impairment. The number of genetic conditions associated with intellectual disabilities is large and increasing, and impossible to commit to memory. You should have a strategy of searching for current information about conditions that are identified in the patients referred to you, and retain a copy of the information in the person's case notes.

Developmental history

Assess and diagnose developmental disorders before reaching a conclusion about the presence or absence of an acquired disorder. Summarize the case by using the headings of a standard psychiatric history, but replace the heading 'personal history' with the phrase 'developmental history' and include information, if available, from the time of conception onwards. It is convenient to add a section on problem behaviours, where you may include information that is sometimes listed as 'habits' such as smoking, and 'forensic history'. Whether or not there is an identifiable developmental disorder, record the person's optimum developmental level. The most suitable way to do this in the standard psychiatric history is to replace the heading 'premorbid personality' with the phrase 'premorbid functioning' and to include information about functioning in all the relevant domains: cognitive, communicative, emotional, social, interpersonal, sexual.

Current social circumstances

This should include information about support plans, such as supported employment or other daytime activities, home-based support and short breaks.

3.7 Involving others in interviews – the role of a third person

Research to validate the PASADD-10 diagnostic interview found that one quarter of diagnosable disorders would have been overlooked if the person with intellectual disability had not been interviewed, and a similar proportion if there had been no informant [4]. Conduct the interview initially with the patient, asking the informant only to assist the person with reminders. It is important to ensure that the informant has the required information. It is usually futile to ask daytime support workers to describe the person's sleep pattern or to ask a residential support worker about the person's academic attainments. It is often assumed that parents can provide a developmental history, but this may not be reliable. Discrepancies of recall of six months or more in reported developmental milestones were found in 20% of parents of developmentally disabled children by the time children were five years old [5]. Some informants have difficulty distinguishing between their observations and their interpretations. It is essential that an objective description of behaviour is recorded before any attempt is made to analyse its function.

Patients who are unable to provide information when they have not prepared for the interview may nevertheless learn how to give information if they are taught (e.g. how to keep a sleep diary) and another role for a third person is to act as an instructor between interviews, in order to help the person to provide better information.

3.8 Examination

Objective examination of a person's physical and mental functioning should be undertaken using the same approach as for the rest of the population. The main difference is the expected frequency of abnormalities. Be alert to features that may be signs of the following conditions:

- developmental motor disorders (e.g. cerebral palsy, Tourette's syndrome)

- disorders of attention (e.g. ADHD)

- seizure disorders including non-epileptic seizures

- delirium

- adverse drug reactions.

When you are recording your examination, the standard headings of physical examination and mental state examination should be used, but use tests of cognitive function that are valid for the level of developmental ability of the person. Some tests routinely used to identify and monitor progress of dementia, such as the Mini Mental State Examination, have not been validated for this population (and rely on assumptions about educational attainment that are not likely to be valid).

Psychiatrists should make an effort to separate their observations from their interpretations, and record both. For example, avoid recording abnormalities of semantics, syntax and the rate of speech as 'formal thought disorder' or 'flight of ideas' depending on whether you have already interpreted the abnormality as representing schizophrenia or mania. Subsequent reinterpretation is difficult.

Biological investigations

Physical illnesses are important differential diagnoses for most psychiatric presentations in people with intellectual disabilities because of non-specific presentations and the higher prevalence of physical illness compared to other population groups. Full blood count, measures of thyroid, kidney and liver function and blood glucose are important routine blood tests as part of psychiatric assessment, and electroencephalography (EEG) and brain imaging may be indicated where an epileptic disorder, or intracranial pathology need to be investigated as potential causes for psychiatric presentations.

Clinical assessment tools

Adaptive behaviour

The Vineland Adaptive Behaviour Scales are useful for assessing a person's developmental level [6]. They include domains of communication, daily living skills, socialization and motor skills. There is an optional scale for maladaptive behaviour. Information is obtained from an informant who has known the person sufficiently well to report on their ability to perform the activities listed. Brief training is required to use the instrument, which is suitable for any professional in a service for people with intellectual disabilities, such as a nurse or social worker.

Psychiatric symptoms

A well validated tool, the PASADD checklist, [7] is designed for carers to complete and has a role in the screening and monitoring of progress of mental disorders in people with intellectual disabilities. Another version, the Mini-PASADD, may be used by professionals with some competence in conducting assessments (either in mental health or intellectual disability services) [8]. The Mini-PASADD provides a glossary description for a range of psychopathology and is a convenient way of recording a preliminary assessment, or to provide a complementary approach to a focused assessment.

Other tools

Tools to support assessment of risk are becoming available and discussed in Chapter 9. Psychological assessment may be valuable. Applied behavioural analysis (description of the form and function of behaviour) is the basis for providing guidance on behavioural management, and described in detail in Chapter 9. Measurement of declining cognitive function is particularly difficult because the tools used in the general population usually assume premorbid functioning at a higher level than many people with intellectual disabilities attain. The routine clinical tests of concentration and memory that are taught as part of the mental state examination must be adapted and usually have to be individualized in order to reflect what the person prefers to attend to, and what they use their memory for (see Chapter 9).

References

1. Goldberg, D. and Huxley, P. (1980) *Mental Illness in the Community: The Pathway to Psychiatric Care*, Tavistock Publications, London.
2. Wing, J.K., Cooper, J.E. and Sartorius, N. (1974) *Measurement and Classification of Psychiatric Symptoms: An Instruction Manual for the PSE and Catego Program*, Cambridge University Press, London.
3. Royal College of Psychiatrists (2001) *DC-LD: Diagnostic Criteria for Psychiatric Disorders for Use with Adults with Learning Disabilities/Mental Retardation*, Occasional Paper 48, Gaskell Press, London.
4. Moss, S.C., Prosser, H., Ibbotson, B. and Goldberg, D.P. (1996) Respondent and informant accounts of psychiatric symptoms in a sample of patients with learning disability. *Journal of Intellectual Disability Research*, **40**, 457–465.
5. Majnemer, A. and Rosenblatt, B. (1994) Reliability of parental recall of developmental milestones. *Pediatric Neurology*, **10** (44), 304–308.
6. Sparrow, S.S. and Cicchetti, D.V. (1985) Diagnostic uses of the Vineland Adaptive Behavior Scales. *Journal of Pediatric Psychology*, **10**, 215–225.
7. Moss, S.C., Prosser, H., Costello, H. *et al.* (1998) Reliability and validity of the PAS-ADD Checklist for detecting psychiatric disorders in adults with intellectual disability. *Journal of Intellectual Disability Research*, **42**, 173–183.
8. Prosser, H., Moss, S.C., Costello, H. *et al.* (1998) Reliability and validity of the Mini PAS-ADD for assessing psychiatric disorders in adults with intellectual disability. *Journal of Intellectual Disability Research*, **42**, 264–272.

Further reading and useful resources

Guidance for communicating with people with intellectual disabilities is provided by several voluntary and public service organizations. Some of the 'Books beyond words' series are useful for referrers and carers to explain what to expect when meeting a doctor (available through the Royal College of Psychiatrists at http://www.rcpsych.ac.uk/publications/booksbeyondwords.aspx).

DC-LD [3] (diagnostic criteria for psychiatric disorders for use with adults with learning disabilities/mental retardation) uses a biopsychosocial-developmental model closely related to ICD-10, which allows diagnoses using ICD-10 if sufficient information is available, and permits less specific descriptions and provisional diagnoses to be made in cases where less information can be obtained. Useful guidance for assessing mental ill health of people with moderate to profound intellectual disabilities is included, such as suggested questions for assessing psychotic symptoms.

More detailed advice about assessing mental ill health may be found at

(http://www.intellectualdisability.info/mental_phys_health/classification_ac.html)

4 Assessing Mental Capacity and Making Best Interest Decisions

Ian Hall and Afia Ali
East London NHS Foundation Trust, UK

4.1 Introduction

Many people with intellectual disability can make many decisions for themselves and should be encouraged to do so. However, some people, particularly those with moderate to severe intellectual disabilities, are unable to make decisions particularly if the decision is complex. Many countries now have legal frameworks and legislation for dealing with situations where people lack capacity. Because we cannot cover all jurisdictions comprehensively, we have used as an example the law in England and Wales, and drawn out general principles for approaching the issue of mental capacity and making best interest decisions where appropriate.

The English and Welsh Mental Capacity Act 2005 [1] provides the statutory framework to enable people lacking capacity to make decisions for themselves or for others to act on the person's behalf. Its accompanying code of practice [2] provides clear guidance on how to apply the principles of the Act in practice.

The Act covers a range of decisions or acts that may be carried out on behalf of someone lacking capacity from everyday decision making such as what to wear, to life changing decisions such as whether to move to a care home or to have a major operation. However, there are certain decisions that the Act does not cover. These include decisions such as consenting to sexual intercourse, and consenting to marriage, divorce or a civil partnership (for same sex couples). Similarly, if a person

Intellectual Disability Psychiatry: a practical handbook   Angela Hassiotis, Diana Andrea Barron and Ian Hall (eds)
© 2009 John Wiley & Sons, Ltd

is detained under the legislation for the treatment of mental disorder (in England and Wales the Mental Health Act 1983 as amended [3]), the Mental Capacity Act does not cover decisions relating to consent and treatment for a mental disorder as these are governed by the Mental Health Act.

There are five core principles in the Mental Capacity Act that govern practice in England and Wales, and are a reflection of good practice generally.

- The most fundamental principle is that people (over the age of 16) are presumed to be able to make decisions for themselves unless it can be shown that they lack capacity to do so. Some people may be able to make decisions for themselves but require assistance to communicate their decision. This does not mean that they cannot make the decision.

- The second principle requires that all practical steps are taken to help a person make a decision before concluding that they lack capacity.

- Thirdly, a person who has capacity is free to make any decision they wish, even if this decision appears unwise. Each individual has their own values, attitudes and preferences, which should be respected, even if they differ from our own.

- The fourth principle states that anything that is done on behalf of someone lacking capacity should be in the person's best interests and not the best interests of, for example family members or professionals. Exceptions to this principle are when an advance decision to refuse treatment has been made, or for example during research, where other safeguards apply.

- The fifth principle states that when making decisions for, or performing acts on a person lacking capacity, consideration should be given to those that are less likely to impinge on the person's human rights and freedoms – 'the least restrictive alternative'. However, sometimes it will be necessary to select an option that is not the least restrictive, if it is in the person's best interests.

4.2 Assessment of capacity

Capacity is 'decision-specific': it is the ability of a person to make a specific decision at the time that it needs to be made. Capacity may fluctuate over time, for example in the case of delirium, or during the course of a relapse of a mental illness. A person may have the capacity to make some more straightforward decisions such as what to eat or what to wear, and not for other more complex decisions such as where to live or whether to have a medical procedure.

Capacity should be assessed by the person responsible for a particular aspect of care or treatment. For decisions about medical treatment, it is ultimately the responsibility of the clinician in charge of that treatment to make a decision regarding someone's capacity. Psychiatrists may feel confident in assessing capacity, but general practitioners, physicians or surgeons may wish to consult others, or to get a second opinion about capacity and whether decision making ability may improve over time.

Decisions about the day-to-day care of someone lacking capacity are usually made by carers. Family members and paid carers do not have to make a formal assessment of capacity but they must take 'reasonable steps' to show that the person lacks the capacity to make a particular decision. In decisions relating to matters of law, it is usually necessary for the person's solicitor or the court to make an assessment, for example, for litigation capacity, and expert psychiatric advice may be sought to assist this.

There are two stages in determining whether someone lacks capacity: Firstly it must be established that there is 'an impairment of, or disturbance in the functioning of, the mind or brain'. This can include organic brain pathology such as dementia, delirium, stroke, head injury and some people with intellectual disabilities. It can also include more 'functional' psychiatric conditions such as depression, schizophrenia and even substance misuse. The second part of the test is that the impairment or disturbance is sufficient to affect their judgement and ability to make a decision. For someone to have capacity, the following four criteria must be met:

1. He/she must be able to understand the information relevant to the decision; and
2. retain the information; and
3. use the information in the process of making the decision; and
4. communicate the decision (by any means).

It is therefore crucial in the assessment of capacity to determine what information is relevant to the particular decision in question. This includes the nature of the decision, why the decision needs to be made, and the likely effects of deciding one way or another, or not making the decision at all. The person must be able to retain the information long enough in order to make the decision. Retention of information may be facilitated through the use of, for example, notebooks, photographs, DVDs or voice recorders. The person must also be able to use the information in order to arrive at the decision and be able to communicate their decision. If the person has difficulties communicating, steps should be taken to facilitate their communication (see below).

A person is considered to be lacking capacity to make a decision if they are unable to perform at least one of the above. Thus, if they are unable to explain the risks or benefits of a recommended procedure even after explanation, or unable to recall information presented to them, or have an irrational explanation for arriving at a decision (e.g. based on persecutory delusions or suicidal ideation), or are unable to communicate because of brainstem injury or a comatose state, then they do not have capacity. If asked to advise physicians and surgeons about a person's decision making ability, it is crucial to work with them to determine the information relevant to the decision. If capacity is borderline it is helpful to reduce this information to the minimum necessary, as presenting too much information can impair decision making.

Helping people to make decisions

A number of strategies can be employed to help people with intellectual disabilities make decisions for themselves and relates to the second principle of the Act. Firstly, has the person been provided with all the relevant information necessary in order to make a decision, including all the alternative options? However, too much information may confuse the person and so a judgement needs to be made about what amount of detail is appropriate for the individual. There are simple ways that communication can be maximized. Much more detail is provided in the chapter relating to communication (Chapter 2); however, to summarize: it is always necessary to find out what the best way to communicate with the person is. Information should be presented using simple language, and may need to be broken down into smaller chunks and given at an appropriate pace, as he or she may require time to process the information. Some people prefer visual aids or a non-verbal method of communication (e.g. Makaton). It may be necessary to repeat the information several times and to check the person's understanding (e.g. ask them to say what you said in their own words). Family members or staff who know the person well may also be able to support the person to communicate and advocates may be able to help the person express their viewpoint. The person also may prefer a particular setting or a particular time of the day. It is important to be aware of religious and cultural factors that may influence decision making.

Someone with a sensory impairment may require additional aids such as special glasses, hearing aids, voice synthesizers or computer technology to communicate. If English is not the person's first language, always involve an interpreter. One should also always consider whether the decision can be postponed until the person's circumstances change. For example, someone with a psychosis in addition to an intellectual disability may regain capacity following treatment of the psychosis.

In emergency medical situations, it may be necessary to treat the person in their best interests immediately and therefore it may not be possible to take steps to help people make decisions. However, health care staff should attempt to communicate with the person and inform them about what is happening.

If the person does have capacity and refuses an investigation or treatment, their decision should be respected. The outcome of the capacity assessment and their decision should be clearly documented but they should be given the opportunity to change their mind.

Case vignette 4.1 Helping people make decisions

Kevin is a 37-year-old man with Down's syndrome and moderate intellectual disability. He is socially isolated and spends most of his day at home with his elderly mother. His mother would like him to develop some of his basic daily living skills and socialize more with other people. His social worker explores some daytime activities that Kevin could get involved with, such as a day centre, or a voluntary work scheme. Kevin has difficulty understanding the different options. His mother informs the social worker that Kevin has not had a health check-up for many years. Physical examination reveals that Kevin has bilateral conductive hearing loss due to a build up of ear wax, which is treated with ear syringing. An improvement in his hearing, in combination with visual aids, makes it easier for Kevin to consider the different options available to him. He still has difficulty deciding so his social worker arranges for Kevin to visit the placements with his mother and, after several visits, Kevin decides that he would like to attend the day centre.

4.3 Making best interest decisions

Case vignette 4.2 Making welfare decisions for someone lacking capacity

Sebastian is a 19-year-old male with a mild intellectual disability. He moved to the UK with his mother two years ago from Nigeria after his parents separated. Sebastian has been living with his mother in a hostel after they were evicted from their flat following rent arrears. His mother works at a local supermarket during the day and leaves Sebastian on his own for long periods of time. Sebastian has few independent living skills and requires assistance with most activities including preparing simple meals. He is not allowed to go out on his own and rarely leaves the hostel. His mother leaves him plain bread and water to eat. He is afraid to use the communal toilet and therefore urinates into a bucket, which his mother cleans. His mother has a tendency to hoard items and therefore the room they live in is occupied by piles of paper and old furniture and there is little room to move around. Sebastian sits on a chair all day long and his only source of entertainment is a radio. Concerns were raised about Sebastian's well-being by the hostel managers, resulting in the local intellectual disability team attempting to engage with Sebastian and his mother. However, his mother prevented social workers and health professionals from gaining access to Sebastian and was frequently verbally abusive towards them. The team were concerned that he was being neglected by his mother and that this was impacting on his physical and mental health. He was underweight and there were signs of malnourishment. However, there were conflicts within the team as to whether he had the capacity to decide whether to accept help from services and to decide where to live.

The team took his case to the Court of Protection. A second opinion was sought on his capacity to make a range of decisions including where to live and what was in his best interests. He was found not to have the capacity to make decisions about his welfare due to his limited understanding, inability to retain information, and inability to weigh up information due to the undue influence that his mother had on him. The professionals working with him felt that it would be in his best interests to be placed in residential care, with supervised visits with his mother, and this was agreed by the court. The court also appointed a deputy to make future decisions on behalf of Sebastian.

Case vignette 4.3   The case of S*

S is an 18-year-old man with velo-cardio-facial syndrome, moderate intellectual disability and autism. As a child, he had had progressively worsening renal failure. In his early teens he presented with end-stage renal failure in an emergency and received emergency haemodialysis but his behaviour was difficult to manage and he needed to be physically restrained. He subsequently settled down, became accustomed to the routine and continued on haemodialysis for several years. As he approached adulthood, the hospital managers took the case to court, arguing that it was not in S's best interests for peritoneal dialysis to be performed and for him to have a renal transplant. They also sought permission to stop haemodialysis and for palliative care to be provided. Their decision was based on the reasoning that S had a fear of needles and therefore haemodialysis was only possible with an indwelling catheter (rather than an aterio-venous fistula, which had lower rates of infection and offered greater freedom). The renal unit felt that the family would find it difficult to cope with peritoneal dialysis and that S also found medical intervention distressing. They did not think that he would be able to cope with the complications of a renal transplant and intensity of visits and blood tests. They also argued that they would not be able to provide the same intensive service as the paediatric unit.

S's parents did not accept that the hospital's plan was in his best interests. They were willing to provide the high level of support that was required of peritoneal dialysis. His mother was willing to donate her kidney and initial tests indicated compatibility.

The court recommended an independent assessment of S's capacity and opinion regarding his best interests. During the independent assessment, S was found to have a relative impairment in his verbal communication but was able to use visual aids and Makaton signs. The renal unit had not attempted to communicate with him using these approaches, and had not involved a speech and language therapist. It was felt that S had the capacity to learn new information using visual aids and if given time. S also appeared to have a good quality of life. He attended school regularly and had activities outside of school such as swimming and enjoyed playing. Although S did not like needles, his previous hospital had successfully used distraction techniques.

Although the court found that S lacked capacity, they acknowledged he could participate more in decision making. The court ruled that it was in his best interests that haemodialysis with a catheter should continue and that peritoneal dialysis should be actively pursued. The court also ruled that haemodialysis with an aterio-venous fistula and renal transplantation should not be excluded on non-medical grounds.

*Taken from a legal court case [4]

If a person lacks capacity, then it may be necessary to make decisions on their behalf, in their best interests (Table 4.1). The Code of Practice to the Mental Capacity Act [2], while not defining 'best interests', gives guidance in the form of a checklist on how to go about making such decisions. Such decisions must always be in the *person*'s best interests (and not e.g. what is in the best interest of the carer or the service provider where there is a conflict). It is important not to discriminate against people or to make value judgements on the basis of their age, appearance, condition or behaviour. In the case of life sustaining treatment, judgements should not be made about whether someone has a good quality of life and decisions should not be motivated by a desire to bring the person's life to an end.

All the circumstances that are relevant to the person should be taken into account as if they were making the decision for themselves. Health professionals may be tempted to take a narrow, medical view of decisions and only take account of factors such as the likelihood of success of a treatment, and the risk of complications. However, other 'welfare' factors are also likely to be relevant, such as effect on activities of daily living, and home life. The person's past and present wishes should be considered, including any verbal requests or requests in writing such as advance decisions. Their religious, cultural or moral beliefs should also be taken into account and those involved in the person's care should also be consulted for their opinion. For those with limited verbal communication, it is especially important to consider non-verbal

Table 4.1   Key steps for determining best interests

---

1. Don't make assumptions.
2. Try to identify all the issues which are most relevant to the person who lacks capacity.
3. Consider whether the person is likely to regain capacity.
4. Do whatever is possible to permit and encourage the person to participate, or to improve his/her ability to participate, as fully as possible in making the decision.
5. Try to find out the views of the person lacking capacity, including:

    a. The person's past and present wishes and feelings.

    b. Both his/her current views and whether the person has expressed any relevant views in the past, either verbally, in writing or through behaviour or habits.

    c. Any beliefs and values (e.g. religious, cultural or moral) that would be likely to influence the decision in question.

    d. Any other factors the person would be likely to consider if able to do so.

6. Consult other people:

    a. Anyone previously named by the person lacking capacity as someone to be consulted.

    b. Carers, close relatives or friends who take an interest in the person's welfare.

    c. Any attorney of a lasting power of attorney made by the person.

    d. Any deputy appointed by the Court of Protection to make decisions for the person.
    Or . . .

    e. independent mental capacity advocate (IMCA): For decisions about major medical treatment or a change of residence and where there is no one who fits into any of the above categories, an IMCA

7. Weigh up all of the above factors in order to determine what decision or course of action is in the person's best interests.

---

expressions of wishes and feelings, both made contemporaneously and in the past. It is usually good practice to hold a best interests meeting with all the parties concerned.

In difficult cases, it may be necessary to get legal advice or to obtain a second opinion. Situations where this may occur include if the person disputes a finding of lack of capacity, or there are disagreements between professionals and family members about the person's capacity or what is in their best interests, if the person expresses different views to different people and if someone is being accused of abusing a vulnerable adult lacking capacity (see Case vignette 4.2).

Case vignette 4.3 describes a real legal case applying the principles of making best interest decisions about medical treatment. This case highlights a number of important points:

- No attempt was made to help S gain capacity by providing information in an accessible way, even though it was known how to communicate optimally with him.

- The importance of acknowledging the views of carers, and communicating effectively with them.

- How easy it is to make judgements about whether someone has a good quality of life based on our own value systems, and the value of taking the time to find out about a person with intellectual disabilities' life circumstances before trying to make medical decisions in their best interests.

Case vignette 4.2 describes a scenario highlighting concerns about the welfare of a person with intellectual disability. In this situation there are concerns that the individual is being neglected by his carer. As the carer is unwilling to cooperate with professionals, and there are disagreements between professionals about whether the person has capacity to make decisions, the case is taken to court.

All decisions and the reason for a particular course of action should be well documented, including any discussions with the individual or their carers. Involving advocates should always be considered, and under the Mental Capacity Act, an independent mental capacity advocates (IMCAs) should be involved for 'unbefriended' people (who have no one to consult apart from a paid carer) regarding decisions about serious medical treatment or where a significant change in residence is being proposed.

Going to court

Most decisions under the Mental Capacity Act can be made without reference to a court. However, the Mental Capacity Act has set up a special court, the Court of Protection with the authority to deal with serious or complex welfare and health care decisions. There are some situations concerning incapacitated people, where it is considered mandatory to make an application to the court. These include situations where there are proposals for life sustaining treatment to be withdrawn in people who are in a persistent vegetative state, where organ or bone marrow donation or non-therapeutic sterilization is being considered and in cases where there may be doubt about whether a treatment is in someone's best interest (e.g. in the Case of S, Case vignette 4.3). Other cases that may be brought to court include disputes about whether a person lacks capacity, disputes between family and professionals and where there may be ethical dilemmas (e.g. innovative treatments).

Court-appointed deputies

In some situations, under the Mental Capacity Act the court can appoint a person (known as a deputy) to act and make decisions on behalf of the person lacking capacity, particularly where a series of decisions need to be made and the person is unlikely to regain capacity for a long time (see Case vignette 4.2).

4.4 Planning for losing capacity

Sometimes people with intellectual disabilities who currently have capacity to make particular decisions may lose capacity in the future, perhaps due to an additional progressive condition like dementia, or a relapsing and remitting one like bipolar disorder.

Adults with capacity can make an *advance decision to refuse treatment* that may be offered to them in the future when they have lost their capacity to consent or refuse treatment. The advance decision must be valid and applicable to current circumstances (e.g. the person must have been aware of current treatment options). Where the decision concerns life sustaining treatment, the decision must be in writing, should be signed and witnessed and it should clearly state that the decision stands even if their life is at risk.

A person with capacity (donor) may authorize another person, an attorney, to make decisions for them regarding welfare (health care and treatment) in their best interests if they lose capacity. An attorney can also be authorized to make decisions for the person regarding property and affairs, including financial matters, although the donor does not have to lack capacity. Such a *lasting power of attorney* (LPA) is a legal document that permits another person to act on the person's behalf. Separate LPAs must be made for decisions regarding welfare and property and affairs. For it to be valid, it must be registered with the Public Guardian. The attorney can accept or refuse medical examination or treatment on the person's behalf. An attorney does not have the right to refuse consent to life saving treatment, unless it is explicitly authorized within the LPA document.

4.5 Deprivation of liberty safeguards

Case vignette 4.4   The 'Bournewood' ruling

H.L., a man with autism and intellectual disability who lacked capacity to make decisions about treatment, was admitted to Bournewood Hospital under the common law doctrine of 'necessity' following an episode of self-harm. He did not object to the admission and therefore the Mental Health Act (MHA) 1983 was not applied. Legal proceedings were brought against the hospital by his paid carers who claimed that he had been unlawfully detained. The claim was rejected by the High Court, which stated that the detention was in his best interests and therefore lawful. The Court of Appeal disagreed with this decision as it believed that the detention would have been lawful if he had been detained under the MHA 1983. The decision was reversed by the House of Lords.

The case was then taken to the European Court of Human Rights. In October 2004, it found that H.L.'s detention under the common law contravened article 5(1) 'the right to liberty' as it lacked sufficient safeguards, such as those that were available under the MHA 1983, and it also infringed article 5(4), the right for a person's detention to be reviewed speedily by the court. The court ruled that the judicial review proceedings were inadequate to meet the requirements of article 5(4).

Sometimes it is necessary to deprive people who lack capacity of their liberty for the purposes of care or the treatment of a physical or mental disorder, in their best interests. Following the Bournewood ruling, [5] the European Court of Human Rights has upheld that when this happens, there needs to be a legal process governing it (see Case vignette 4.4). As a result of this, new safeguards have been introduced to the Mental Capacity Act [6] to protect people in these circumstances, with a formal process of assessment and authorization. The safeguards apply to people in hospitals and care homes, and cover a range of situations where someone's liberty could be deprived such as the use of restraint and sedation, restrictions on a person's social contacts and loss of autonomy because a person is under constant supervision and control by members of staff. The authorization is just for the deprivation of liberty – any other aspect of medical treatment or other care provided in someone's best interests is governed by the main Mental Capacity Act provisions.

There are six criteria to determine whether deprivation of liberty is appropriate. These are formally assessed by specially trained mental health assessors and best interest assessors:

1. The person must be 18 years of age or over.
2. There are no valid refusals or conflicts with an existing authority to make decisions (e.g. advance decision or a valid decision of a donee or deputy).
3. The person lacks capacity.
4. The person has a disorder or disability of the mind or brain.
5. The person is eligible (not subject to detention under the Mental Health Act, and there is no conflict with the community provisions of the Mental Health Act).
6. The deprivation of liberty must be in the best interests of the person.

The deprivation of liberty safeguards are not appropriate if the person objects to being treated in hospital for mental disorder. In this situation, it may be necessary to detain the person under the Mental Health Act, if this applies.

4.6 The use of the Mental Health Act

The Mental Capacity Act can be used to treat physical disorders in people lacking capacity, and enables the treatment of mental disorders that might need to be treated outside of a psychiatric hospital, for example less severe mental illnesses that can be treated in community settings, and disorders with a physical basis such as delirium and temporal lobe status that may be treated in general hospitals. However, where its powers are required, the Mental Health Act should be used to provide the authority to treat, particularly where there are issues related to deprivation of liberty. The Mental Health Act can be used in the treatment of mental disorders and their physical causes or consequences such as self-harm secondary to depression, or treating Cushing's syndrome-induced psychosis.

4.7 Conducting research with people who lack capacity

There is no doubt that in the past research was carried out inappropriately on people who lack capacity, such as the radiation experiments on children with intellectual disabilities at the Walter E. Fernald State School in Massachusetts between 1946 and 1953 [7].

The Mental Capacity Act and its Code of Practice [2] provide guidelines about conducting research with people lacking capacity, in order to protect vulnerable individuals from abuse or exploitation. In England and Wales, ethical approval must be obtained before research can be conducted. The research must relate to the condition that is the cause of the person's impairment or the treatment of that condition. There must be reasonable grounds for believing that the research cannot be effectively conducted with people who have capacity, and that steps have been taken to consult carers and other people involved in the person's care. In addition, the research must either benefit the person in some way (but benefits must be weighed up against risks), or provide knowledge about the cause, treatment or care of the person's condition (but risks must be negligible, and should not interfere with their freedom and be restrictive). Any objections that a person lacking capacity makes during the research should be noted and respected.

4.8 Children and young people

The Mental Capacity Act does not apply to children below the age of 16. Most of the Act applies to young people aged 16 and 17 with the exception that only people over the age of 18 can make a LPA and can make an advance decision to refuse medical treatment. There is a lot of overlap with legislation governing children (e.g. the Children's Act 1989 [8]) and no specific rules about when to apply which Act. Difficulties may arise if a young person has capacity to make a decision and refuses treatment, especially if someone with parental responsibility disagrees with this decision and wishes to provide consent on the person's behalf. Such disputes may need to be settled by the Family Division of the High Court (and not the Court of Protection). Currently under common law, a person with parental responsibility can consent to the young person receiving medical treatment if they lack capacity. However, health care professionals can provide treatment or care providing it is in the person's best interests, whether or not parental consent is obtained. Every effort should be taken to consult those involved in the person's care, although confidentiality should be respected.

4.9 Conclusion

For professionals and carers looking after people with intellectual disabilities, the most important development in legislation in England and Wales is the Mental Capacity Act. This has put into statute a clear process for determining people's capacity to make decisions, what to do if people lack capacity, and provisions for people who may lose capacity to make decisions in the future. It provides safeguards for people who may be deprived of their liberty, or who are subjected to abusive practices. A clear role for community intellectual disability services is to support other professionals such as general practitioners, hospital doctors and carers in their role in assessing capacity to make decisions for which they are responsible, and in making best interest decisions for those who lack capacity. The principles of maximizing communication, considering the views of carers and the values and beliefs and wishes of the patient (even if they lack capacity) are all highly relevant.

References

1. Mental Capacity Act 2005, The Stationery Office, London.
2. Department for Constitutional Affairs (2007) *Code of Practice. Mental Capacity Act 2005*, The Stationery Office, London.
3. Mental Health Act 2007, The Stationery Office, London.
4. (2003) An Hospital NHS Trust and S (by his litigation friend the Official Solicitor and DG (S's father) and SG (S's mother). In the High Court of Justice, Family Division: Neutral Citation No: [2003] EWHC 365 (Fam).
5. *H.L. vs United Kingdom*, no 45508/99, ECHR 2004 – IX.
6. Ministry of Justice (2008) *Mental Capacity Act 2005: Deprivation of Liberty Safeguards: Code of Practice to Supplement the Main Mental Capacity Act 2005 Code of Practice*, The Stationery Office, London.

7. United States Department of Energy (1994) Advisory Committee on Human Radiation, Part II, Chapter 7.
8. The Children Act 1989, The Stationery Office, London.

Further reading

Department for Constitutional Affairs (2007) *Code of Practice. Mental Capacity Act 2005*, The Stationery Office.

Department of Health (2008) *Code of Practice. Mental Health Act 1983*, The Stationery Office, London.

Department of Health (2008) *Reference Guide to the Mental Health Act 1983*, The Stationery Office, London.

5 Common Mental Disorders (Depression, Anxiety, OCD, PTSD)

Elspeth Bradley[1], Rebecca Goody[2], Shirley McMillan[3] and
Andrew Levitas[4]

[1]*Department of Psychiatry, University of Toronto, Canada*
[2]*Cornwall Partnership NHS Trust, UK*
[3]*Surrey Place Centre, Toronto, Canada*
[4]*Department of Psychiatry, University of Medicine and Dentistry, New Jersey, USA*

5.1 Introduction

Persons with intellectual disabilities, across the ability range, experience mood and anxiety disturbances and for some, clinically significant disorders may arise. Overall the prevalence of mood disorders is at least the same and for anxiety disorders (e.g. phobic disorders) even greater than in the general population [1, 2]. The consistently high rate of behaviour problems identified in this population [3] may point to unrecognized anxiety and mood disturbances associated with these behaviour problems; mental health professionals not trained to worked with this population may be under-diagnosing these conditions [4, 5]. The negative impact such mood and anxiety disturbances have on individuals with intellectual disabilities give rise to additional functional disabilities and physical disorders, poor health, further exclusion from mainstream activities and social opportunities and poorer quality of life. Mental health professionals working with people with intellectual disabilities are privileged in having the opportunity to guide and participate in the prevention of such negative outcomes.

Intellectual Disability Psychiatry: a practical handbook   Angela Hassiotis, Diana Andrea Barron and Ian Hall (eds)
© 2009 John Wiley & Sons, Ltd

5.2 Anxiety

Anxiety is a normal experience alerting the person to some impending danger so that an appropriate adaptive response can be made. Stress is experienced when an event overwhelms individual resources and coping strategies. In typical development, increasing cognitive and communicative skills and abilities empower the individual to optimally manage ongoing, or anticipated, anxiety and stress. Prior to developing these skills, the person relies on others to anticipate, modulate and minimize stressful situations and to assist in managing anxiety and stress when these occur. Adults with intellectual disabilities will have different capacities in these regards. In working with adults with intellectual disabilities it is important therefore to:

- Identify each adult's developmental capacity to understand and manage anxiety and stress.

- Assist carers to build structures and supports necessary to (i) reduce exposure for that adult to unnecessary stressful situations, and (ii) promote resilience in that adult to handle anxiety and stress across the lifespan (e.g. carer understanding of client's emotional and communication needs, skill-enhancement-based supports, psychological therapies).

Case vignette 5.1   Anxiety

Adam, 25 years, with fragile X syndrome, would, in response to upsets (e.g. disappointment, overstimulating environments), suddenly become agitated, appear nervous and pick up whatever was around and wave this provocatively and dangerously at others. Because of his unpredictability in these regards, he was unable to travel alone to and from work. Anxiolytic medication had not been helpful. Carers were taught about fragile X syndrome including the associated sensory sensitivities, high arousal and social anxiety. With Adam's assistance the behaviour therapist helped staff recognize Adam's escalating anxiety, agitation and distress along an escalation behaviour continuum and identified strategies to support him at these times. Staff then helped Adam recognize his own internal experience of increasing anxiety and supported him in de-escalation strategies (e.g. cognitive behaviour therapy and controlled relaxation). This learning was facilitated by using visual scripts, verbal and non-verbal controlling signals. Beta blockers were successful in reducing his physiological arousal and psychological experience of distress. Over several months of this support Adam was able to travel to work on his own without incident. However, with each change of staff in his home, reports of behaviour incidents travelling home from work, which sometimes involved police support, would increase. These incidents would again diminish once these new staff took part in education about fragile X syndrome and training to support Adam in recognizing and managing his own anxiety.

5.3 Mood

The experience of mood is a sustained and pervasive feeling tone that influences the person's behaviour and perception of the world, the external expression of which is affect. *Affect regulation* refers to the capacity to regulate mood and affective expression in response to internal and external experiences. Healthy people experience a wide range of moods and are observed to have an equally wide range of affective expressions: essentially they feel in control of their moods and affects. Affect regulation is a process that starts from birth and is greatly influenced through the experience of early attachments. People with intellectual disabilities have different capacities to describe their moods and other emotional states, and how they feel pain and other bodily discomforts; these capacities are greatly enhanced by communication assistance and support, leading to improved physical health and emotional well being. Some points of note are shown in Box 5.1.

Box 5.1   Mood-important points

- Some syndromes are associated with problems in affect regulation (e.g. autism spectrum disorders (ASD)). For others with intellectual disabilities, early separations and experiences (e.g. institutional living) have resulted in disruption of attachments and consequent problems in affect regulation. These adults are particularly vulnerable to mood disturbance and negative subjective experiences and evaluation of themselves.

- A sense of being held positively in the regard of others (feeling valued and respected) along with involvement in meaningful and purposeful activities are powerful mood enhancing experiences.

- Recognizing these disturbances in affect regulation and their origins offers opportunities for the prevention of mood disorders and more successful treatment when these occur.

Case vignette 5.2 Mood

Mona, 15 years, was adopted at 18 months having suffered neglect whilst living with her biological mother and then physical abuse in foster care. She had a history of deafness from recurrent ear infections, was severely underweight when adopted and during her childhood had several painful procedures associated with skeletal abnormalities. She thrived, however, living with her adoptive parents who were very intuitive to her intellectual disabilities needs and, despite being somewhat of a perfectionist, Mona was able to experience success in her school work and positive self-esteem with her peers.

In the two years following her mother being hospitalized for major surgery, Mona suffered three discrete episodes of dramatic behaviour change, lasting one to two weeks each. During these episodes she showed: loss of skills, weight loss, had to be fed, her sleep was disrupted, she was unable to engage in previously loved activities, appeared confused and disoriented (more than depressed or sad) and at times appeared anxious and was self-blaming. The episodes typically started suddenly over a 24–48 hour period and ended equally suddenly but taking two or three days before she returned to full functioning. Selective serotonin reuptake inhibitor medication was started after the second episode, but did not prevent the third episode occurring some months later. Despite extensive physical investigations no physical cause for these episodes of changed behaviour was found.

In the absence of such, the community intellectual disabilities team considered Mona's episodes could be understood as her experience of helplessness and overwhelming emotional response to the 'loss' of her adoptive mother (due to hospitalization and subsequent incapacities) in being able to provide much needed physical and emotional supports, awakening earlier such experiences in infancy and childhood. Mona started with a psychotherapist experienced in working with adolescents with intellectual disabilities. Two years on Mona has not had any further 'episodes' despite her mother again requiring further surgery. She and her family report pleasure in her current achievements. She is no longer on medication.

5.4 Aetiological considerations

People with intellectual disabilities represent a small sub-group within the general population and therefore the aetiological circumstances giving rise to mood and anxiety disturbances in the general population will also apply to those with intellectual disabilities [6]. However, the aetiological circumstances giving rise to intellectual disabilities (e.g. brain damage and psychosocial adversity) and the daily impact of intellectual disabilities, for example trying to participate in everyday activities without needed supports and adaptations, also need to be considered in the development and maintenance of mood and anxiety disorders in this group. These latter circumstances may not always be sufficiently appreciated in the psychiatric diagnostic formulation, treatment and care plan for the patient with intellectual disability in mainstream mental health services. This can give rise to heroic, but unsuccessful diagnostic and treatment efforts if the professionals do not acknowledge the extent to which the psychosocial, developmental and habilitative supports have to be put in place before the more traditional psychiatric treatment and care is effective. As a result, people with intellectual disabilities can be left over-medicated, under-treated and marginalized within generic mental health services.

Additional reasons contributing to anxiety and mood disturbances in the population with intellectual disabilities include the following:

- Medical – syndrome-related medical disorders – for example thyroid problems in Down syndrome; greater prevalence of seizures; greater prevalence of undiagnosed medical conditions; other disabilities (e.g. hearing, vision, motor) that interfere with daily activities; greater use of psychotropic medications giving rise to side effects.

- Trauma/abuse (higher prevalence of physical, sexual and emotional abuse).

- Poor adaptive coping skills.

- Poor problem solving abilities.

- Cognitive deficits, particularly temporal memory, can influence how people with intellectual disabilities experience life events leading them to experience historical events in distorted timescales [7].

- Heightened and different sensory sensitivities may be more prevalent in some conditions, for example autism spectrum disorder.

- Loss of significant others are associated with out-of-home placements, changing care providers, siblings leaving home, aging parents.

- Syndromes with associated mood (e.g. Down, Prader-Willi) and anxiety (e.g. Williams, fragile X, autism spectrum) disturbances.

- Brain damage (e.g. frontal lobe disorders) giving rise to the intellectual disabilities and/or additional damage resulting from associated behaviours (e.g. self-injurious behaviour).

- Diet and lifestyle: higher rates of poor nutrition and inactivity are associated with living arrangements and socio-economic circumstances.

- Stressors: people with intellectual disabilities have less control over their lives and decisions made are less focused on their individual needs.

- Previous unsatisfactory relationships with service providers experienced by the person and/or their family.

5.5 Diagnosing anxiety and mood disorders in people with intellectual disabilities

Concerns as to the applicability of ICD-10 and DSM-IV-TR [8, 9] in diagnosing psychiatric disorders in persons with intellectual disabilities, particularly in those with more severe cognitive and communication disabilities and other associated handicaps (e.g. sensory and motor) have given rise to the Diagnostic Criteria for Psychiatric Disorders for Use with Adults with Learning Disabilities/Mental Retardation (DC-LD) [10], a modified approach based on the ICD system and the Diagnostic Manual-Intellectual Disability (DM-ID) [11], an adaptation of the DSM system. These modifications include helpful descriptions of symptoms and behaviours that may represent mood and anxiety disturbances specific to persons with intellectual disabilities, that is 'atypical' presentations. As such, familiarity with both diagnostic systems and the rich descriptive clinical material contained in these manuals are recommended as invaluable resources to the health professional working with people with intellectual disabilities and mental disorders.

However, the overlap in both aetiological circumstances and psychopathology between anxiety and mood disorders means that sub-typing these disorders for persons with intellectual disabilities is often even more difficult and sometimes remains uncertain. In such circumstances an intervention trial based on targeting key symptoms and behaviours may help elucidate the underlying condition.

The DM-ID assigns a chapter each to obsessive-compulsive disorder (OCD) and post-traumatic stress disorder (PTSD) (which in the DSM-IV-TR appear in the chapter on anxiety disorders) noting the importance of these disorders in the population with intellectual disabilities and the observation that in this population they are frequently under-diagnosed.

The DC-LD provides a hierarchical approach to diagnosis within three main axes:

Axis I: severity of learning disabilities;

Axis II: cause of intellectual disabilities; and

Axis III: psychiatric disorders

with separate levels for developmental disorders (Level A), psychiatric illness (Level B), personality disorders (Level C), problem behaviours (Level D) and other disorders (Level E), in Axis III. This hierarchical approach assists in teasing out the psychiatric and other health comorbidities that frequently occur for persons with intellectual disabilities.

Case vignette 5.3 Atypical presentation

Peter, 32 years, became known to the community intellectual disabilities service two years after the death of his father. He was an only child, and after leaving school worked with his father in a local pizza business answering the telephone. His father died suddenly and Peter lost his job as other employees were not as prepared to support him in answering the telephone. He became moody and his eating erratic; he would spend long hours in his bedroom at home living with his mother and when not there would wander out at night, sometimes ending up in the A&E department having swallowed small objects such as small stones and metal tags. Peter had no explanation for this behaviour and denied any feelings of sadness but would sometimes volunteer he missed his father. Subsequent investigations and assessments showed Peter to have mild intellectual disability and he scored in the autism range in the social and communication parts of the Autism Diagnostic Interview. Upper gastrointestinal investigations showed evidence of acid reflux. He denied any pain or discomfort from this but was observed to cough and gag on his food at times and occasionally would acknowledge fluid coming into his throat when he would stoop to tie his shoe laces. He also showed tics, obsessive thoughts (wanting to break light bulbs) and compulsive behaviours (compulsive buying and destroying video games). These latter behaviours, as well as mood disturbance, were targeted for monitoring over several months and during trials of medication. It was observed that when Peter would become depressed or there was re-emergence of his oesophagitis there was an increase in his visiting the A&E having swallowed small objects.

5.6 Psychiatric assessment of anxiety and mood disorders

The clinical assessment and how to communicate with individuals with intellectual disabilities is discussed in Chapters 2 and 3. In the UK, prior to commencing any assessment or treatment there need to be considerations about capacity to consent [12] (also see Chapter 4). The psychiatric evaluation of the patient with intellectual disability, while similar in some ways to that carried out with the general population, is generally more complex, takes longer and is best done within a multidisciplinary framework (see Appendix B) to enable medical, psychological, communication, sensory and other assessments leading to the development of a more coherent psychiatric diagnostic formulation. This additional complexity arises because:

- The presenting complaints, while initially appearing as mood and anxiety disturbances, may be due to circumstances other than anxiety or mood disorders. A systematic review of all possible contributing or causative factors is therefore required and includes consideration of the following: [13]

  - Biological and medical

  - Expectations on individual

  - Supports and adaptations available

  - Emotional factors

  - Psychiatric disorder.

- The person with intellectual disability may have other clinically significant symptoms, some of which may meet symptom and behavioural criteria for other psychiatric disorders; for example, one, or a combination, of inattention, hyperactivity, impulsivity, obsessional thoughts, compulsive behaviours, phobias, motor and vocal tics and self-injurious behaviours may have been present before the onset of the new concerns. Differentiating between established older symptoms from new onset ones is necessary: [14]

  - to identify the nature of (and diagnose) older established behaviours and symptoms, for example tic disorder

  - to identify (and diagnose) new onset disorders, for example manic episodes

  - to determine where the immediate focus of intervention and treatment should be placed, for example treatment of tics or underlying mania

  - to differentiate from pre-existing problems (e.g. tics) any side effects (e.g. abnormal movements) arising from new medications.

- The person's environment including social and emotional supports may need to be assessed so as to determine whether expectations on the individual are appropriate and supports and adaptations available are sufficient.

- It may be necessary to spend time observing the client where he/she lives and works and spends time.

- Time may need to be spent working with carers to 'stabilize' the individual's supports before it can be determined whether the anxiety or other mood symptoms are in response to insufficient supports and inappropriate expectations or because of an underlying psychiatric disorder.

- Structures for carers to monitor target symptoms may be needed in each of the environments in which the person spends time. It may take extra time to teach and assist the person in self-monitoring.

- A determination as to whether the behaviours and symptoms present in the clinical interview represent new psychopathology can be done only with reference to an understanding of the person's usual or baseline ways of behaving and communicating, as well as other co-occurring psychiatric disorder (e.g. attention deficit hyperactivity disorder ADHD or ASD).

- The following approach and questions may be helpful:

  - Enquire as to when the person was last functioning well or at his/her best.

  - Establish a detailed description of the person's adaptive functioning at that time. One way to approach this is to ask about a typical day from getting up in the morning to going to bed at night.

  - Determine how the person's behaviour has changed from this baseline level of functioning in each area previously explored.

  - Identify target behaviours (e.g. sleep, eating, anxiety ratings) for further monitoring to assist in: (i) confirming the provisional clinical diagnosis and (ii) evaluating response to interventions and treatment.

Case vignette 5.4   Multidisciplinary psychiatric assessment

Miriam, 17 years and with Down syndrome, was referred to the community intellectual disabilities team because of pinching and pushing people at school, resulting in her having been suspended on many occasions. This behaviour had been present from an early age but escalated when she moved to high school. Several months before the referral the family doctor had prescribed two different selective serotonin reuptake inhibitors but each was followed by agitated behaviour and sleep disturbance. When seen by the community team, at interview Miriam sat close to her mother, her head often turned away from the interviewer; she appeared sad and withdrawn but showed concern when her mother became upset and tearful when describing her daughter's several suspensions from school. Mother described Miriam as being perfectly herself at home, interacting with family, eating normally, interested in her DVDs and would still take pleasure in preparing the supper table for the family, which she did competently and independently. However, in past months she had been reluctant to go outside of the home, and once out would often refuse to get out of the car; in restaurants which she previously enjoyed, she would keep her coat on, pulling her hood over her head so that her face was hidden. Out of the home she appeared withdrawn, sad and moved slowly.

On psychological assessment Miriam was found to have moderate/severe intellectual disability – of particular note she showed good daily life skills but her academic work was very poor; she was barely able to pick out or write the letters of her name and could not add two single digits. She met criteria for global intellectual disability as well as specific learning disability. Miriam's articulation was very poor. Hearing impairment in both ears had been identified at an early age but she had refused to wear aids and while a frequency modulated system had been recommended at school this never was implemented. ADHD checklists completed by her school teacher indicated impulsiveness and inattention. It was unclear whether this reflected her intellectual disability, specific learning difficulty, hearing impairment or an attention deficit disorder.

The team behaviour therapist visited her school and home and determined that Miriam engaged in pinching and pushing behaviours when she was trying to communicate her needs – in particular when she did not understand what was going on and had been expected to wait too long for assistance. At these times she would also become much more impulsive and unpredictable. Psychological testing identified that Miriam would become very upset and distressed (and start to pinch and push) when she experienced herself failing (the criteria for terminating psychological testing is when the individual starts not to be able to do the tasks). On the other hand, in formal assessment of communication by the speech and language therapist, Miriam was not aware of when she was failing and did not show distressed behaviours even though she showed significant limitations in this area. Reassessment of her hearing showed that Miriam's hearing was reduced by about 60% in each ear and in the classroom situation it was estimated she might have been picking up only about one quarter of the information.

Miriam was started on stimulant medication and a frequency modulation system was installed in her classroom. Her difficulties with academics were addressed and a more vocational-skills-based programme put in place. Her mood improved in school, and she started to enjoy outside-of-the-home activities again. Re-emergence of the referral behaviours became the 'thermometer' against which her school was able to ensure it continued to meet her developmental, medical and communication needs, so preventing further mental health and behavioural disturbances.

5.7 Treatment of anxiety and mood disorders: additional considerations

In the UK the National Institute for Clinical Excellence (NICE) has provided clinical guidelines for the identification, management and treatment of anxiety (panic disorder, with or without agoraphobia and generalized anxiety disorder), PTSD, OCD, depression and bipolar disorder [15]. These guidelines, with adaptations for individuals with greater communication and cognitive impairments, are also appropriate for individuals with intellectual disabilities.

For persons with intellectual disabilities, given the complexities already discussed, a definitive diagnosis of a specific anxiety or mood disorder is often less readily available (see case vignettes). Instead, these complexities are held within a broader diagnostic formulation that recognizes that the same behaviours (e.g. aggression) at different times may represent different aetiologies [13] that need to be reviewed on an ongoing basis and appropriate interventions offered. Where a more definitive diagnosis of a particular anxiety or mood disorder becomes apparent, then treatment as for the general population is appropriate with the following cautions:

- Treatment with medication: start low, go slow and change one medication at a time as there is a higher frequency of idiosyncratic responses to psychotropic drugs.

- Psychological therapies: to be optimally effective these will need to be adapted and possibly supported by others between sessions, according to the individual's cognitive, communication and concentration capacities.

- Multi-modal interventions, for example psychotherapy, sensory therapy, behaviour therapy, stress management, attention to communication and medication may be necessary [16]. Communication between professionals is important.

- Stakeholders, for example client, family, other carers, need to agree the diagnostic formulation and treatment plan and where more than one intervention is being offered, to understand the focus of each intervention. Where different medications are being used simultaneously, the reason for each needs to be explained.

- Clinical relapse may be due to a different cause from the aetiology for which the medications or other interventions are being targeted. It is wise therefore to have a crisis plan mapped out ahead of time in order to address safety and other issues at these times without sabotaging the ongoing treatment for underlying anxiety or mood disorders.

In the UK, health policy states that people with intellectual disabilities should be supported to access mainstream services [17]. A crucial role for the community team, therefore, is in supporting the relevant mainstream services to adapt their approaches to take into consideration the person with intellectual disability. This may be in the form of direct joint working or indirect consultation and training.

5.8 Prevention

This chapter has focused on the vulnerability of persons with intellectual disabilities to anxiety and mood disorders. It is imperative that the development and delivery of clinical services now embrace what is known about preventing and minimizing these disturbances. Proactive and ongoing attention to issues relating to loss, stress (Box 5.2), anxiety, life events and earlier trauma, and transition planning across the lifespan with real and meaningful service choices for individuals and their families are paramount [18].

Box 5.2   Strategies for managing stress

- Exercise

- Good diet

- Rest and relaxation

- Opportunities to talk, laugh, cry with others and to be felt understood

- Opportunities for supportive social networks and satisfying social connections

- The experience of being safe and feeling safe, respected and valued in a community

---

- Appropriate routines

- Meaningful occupations

- Adequate (from client's perspective) preparation for change and transition using strategies tailor-made for the individual's unique communication and cognitive style and capacities

- Behavioural supports including relaxation repertoires and escalation continuums for clients and staff to guide interventions

- Other psychological stress management strategies that are meaningful to person, for example use of concrete materials to support visual imagery and symbolism, building on client's experience to develop meaningful metaphors in therapy.

Equally important is the availability of interdisciplinary approaches and 'capable environments', [19] understanding of the appropriate use of medication, [20, 21] psychological therapies and other treatment strategies in prevention and when problems arise. Concern about the poorer health and mental health status of persons with intellectual disabilities compared to the general population has given rise to greater focus on this population in countries around the world with the development of national policy documents [17, 22]. The UK has incorporated legislation and greater accountability to ensure policy is enacted in a timely manner [23].

The absence of a national policy direction appears to encourage a more crisis-orientated, reactive response to mental health and behavioural problems and use of emergency services [24]. The latter service model, along with unavailable, inappropriate or insufficient supports, can become part of the trauma and negative life events these individuals and their families experience which may contribute further to the development and maintenance of these anxiety and mood disorders. However, mental health professionals, who understand the complex health needs of this population, regardless of the service system in which they find themselves, remain in a unique position to advocate for appropriate preventive, assessment and treatment services for their individual clients.

Acknowledgements

We are indebted to Ms Marika Korossy who provided invaluable library and editorial assistance.

We also thank Neill Simpson for his input in the case vignettes.

References

1. Deb, S., Matthews, T., Thompson, A. and Bouras, N. (2001) *Practice Guidelines for the Assessment and Diagnosis of Mental Health Problems in Adults with Intellectual Disabilities*, Pavilion, Brighton. Also available at: http://www.estiacentre.org/docs/PracticeGuidelines.pdf.

2. (a) Deb, S., Thomas, M. and Bright, C. (2008) Mental disorder in adults with intellectual disability. 1: prevalence of functional psychiatric illness among a community-based population aged between 16 and 64 years. *Journal of Intellectual Disability Research*, **45** (6), 495–505; (b) Deb, S., Thomas, M. and Bright, C. (2008) Mental disorder in adults with intellectual disability. 2: the rate of behaviour disorders among a community-based population aged between 16 and 64 years. *Journal of Intellectual Disability Research*, **45** (6), 506–514.

3. Cooper, S.A. (2007) Mental ill-health in adults with intellectual disabilities: prevalence and associated factors. *British Journal of Psychiatry*, **190**, 27–35.

4. Lunsky, Y., Bradley, E., Durbin, J. and Koegl, C. (2008) A comparison of patients with intellectual disability receiving specialized and general services in Ontario's psychiatric hospitals. *Journal of Intellectual Disability Research*, **52** (2), 1003–1012.

5. Lunsky, Y., Bradley, E., Durbin, J. *et al.* (2006) The clinical profile and service needs of hospitalized adults with mental retardation and a psychiatric diagnosis. *Psychiatric Services*, **57** (1), 77–83.

6. Gelder, M.G., Andreasen, N.C., López Ibor, J.J. and Geddes, J. (2009) *New Oxford Textbook of Psychiatry*, Oxford University Press, Oxford.

7. Willner, P. and Goodey, R. (2006) Interaction of cognitive distortions and cognitive deficits in the formulation and treatment of obsessive-compulsive behaviours in a woman with an intellectual disability. *Journal of Applied Research in Intellectual Disabilities*, **19** (1), 67–73.

8. World Health Organization (1993) The ICD-10 Classification of Mental and Behavioural Disorders: Diagnostic Criteria for Research, World Health Organization, Geneva.

9. American Psychiatric Association, American Psychiatric Association Task Force on DSM-IV (2000) *Diagnostic and Statistical Manual of Mental Disorders DSM-IV-TR*, 4th edn, text revision. American Psychiatric Association, Washington, DC.

10. Royal College of Psychiatrists (2001) *DC-LD: Diagnostic Criteria for Psychiatric Disorders for Use with Adults with Learning Disabilities/Mental Retardation*, Occasional paper (Royal College of Psychiatrists), OP 48, Gaskell Press, London.

11. Fletcher R.J., Loschen E., Stavrakaki C. and First M. (eds) (2007) *DM-ID: Diagnostic Manual-Intellectual Disability: A Clinical Guide Diagnosis of Mental Disorders in Persons with Intellectual Disability*, NADD Press, Kingston.

12. Scott, S., Sampson, Z., Scott, R. and Shepherd, V. (2007) Making Decisions: a Guide for People Who Work in Health and Social Care – Booklet 3, MCIP: Mental Capacity Implementation Programme, London. Available at: http://www.dca.gov.uk/legal-policy/mental-capacity/mibooklets/booklet03.pdf.

13. Bradley E.A. and Hollins S. (2006) Assessment of patients with intellectual disabilities, in *Psychiatric Clinical Skills* (ed. D.S. Goldbloom), Mosby Elsevier, Philadelphia, pp. 235–253.

14. Bradley, E. and Bolton, P. (2006) Episodic psychiatric disorders in teenagers with learning disabilities with and without autism. *British Journal of Psychiatry*, **189** (4), 361–366.

15. National Institute for Health and Clinical Excellence Mental Health and Behavioural Conditions: Clinical Guidelines [Web Page]. Available at http://www.nice.org.uk/guidance/index.jsp?action=byTopic&o=7281&set=true, (Accessed January 2009).

16. Royal College of Psychiatrists (2004) *Psychotherapy and Learning Disability*, Royal College of Psychiatrists, London, Council Report CR 116. Available at: http://www.rcpsych.ac.uk/files/pdfversion/cr116.pdf.

17. Department of Health (2001) Valuing People: A New Strategy for Learning Disability for the 21st Century [Web Page]. Available at http://www.archive.official-documents.co.uk/document/cm50/5086/5086.pdf, (Accessed January 2009).

18. Levitas, A.S. and Gilson, S.F. (2001) Predictable crises in the lives of people with mental retardation. *Mental Health Aspects of Developmental Disabilities*, **4** (3), 89–100.

19. Banks, R., Bush, A., Baker, P. *et al.* (2007) Challenging Behaviour: A Unified Approach, Royal College of Psychiatrists, British Psychological Society and Royal College of Speech and Language Therapists, London, CR 144. Available at: http://www.rcpsych.ac.uk/files/pdfversion/cr144.pdf.

20. Levitas, A. (1997) Laws of psychopharmacology. *Habilitative Mental Healthcare Newsletter*, **16** (4), 67–69.

21. Deb, S., Clarke, D. and Unwin, G. (2006) Using Medication to Manage Behaviour Problems Among Adults with Learning Disability: Quick Reference Guide (QRG) [Web Page]. September 2006; Available at http://www.ld-medication.bham.ac.uk/qrg.pdf, (Accessed January 2009).

22. The Surgeon General (2002) Closing the Gap: A National Blueprint to Improve the Health of Persons with Mental Retardation [Web Page]. Available at http://www.surgeongeneral.gov/topics/mentalretardation/, (Accessed January 2009).

23. Healthcare Commission, UK Cornwall Partnership NHS Trust Lifted Out of Special Measures after Watchdog Releases Progress Report [Web Page]. Available at http://www.healthcarecomission.org.uk/newsandevents/mediacentre/pressreleases.cfm?cit_id=892&FAArea1=customWidgets.content_view_1&usecache=false, (Accessed January 2009).

24. Lunsky, Y., Garcin, N., Morin, D. *et al.* (2007) Mental health services for individuals with intellectual disabilities in Canada: findings from a national survey. *Journal of Applied Research in Intellectual Disabilities*, Special Issue: Dual Diagnosis, **20** (5), 439–447.

6 Psychotic Illness

Angela Hassiotis[1] and Amanda Sinai[2]

[1]Department of Mental Health Sciences, University College London, UK
[2]Camden Learning Disabilities Service, London, UK

6.1 Introduction

A psychotic disorder is a type of mental disorder that reflects a detachment from reality. It often involves abnormalities in behaviour, speech, thought content and form and insight. Psychotic illnesses can vary from a short-lived episode, which resolves spontaneously, to a chronic disorder, such as schizophrenia.

The prevalence of psychotic symptoms in adults with intellectual disabilities is higher than that of the general population [1]. Assessment, diagnosis and management of psychosis in adults with intellectual disabilities should follow a similar format to that in adults without an intellectual disability. This format may be easier to apply to those with mild intellectual disabilities. As with all cases, it is important to tailor the assessment and management to the individual.

Adults with moderate or severe/profound intellectual disabilities are more likely to have communication difficulties and/or cognitive difficulties, which may pose particular challenges in assessment. In an adult with limited verbal communication, assessment will need to focus on supporting verbal and non-verbal communication, as well as detailed observation of behaviour (including behaviours in different settings), and a thorough collateral history.

This chapter will explore some of the important considerations required when assessing, diagnosing and managing an adult with intellectual disability and a psychotic illness.

Intellectual Disability Psychiatry: a practical handbook   Angela Hassiotis, Diana Andrea Barron and Ian Hall (eds)
© 2009 John Wiley & Sons, Ltd

6.2 Definition

ICD-10 [2] and DSM-IV [3] are international classifications that are used to categorize mental illness. They are often used in adults without intellectual disabilities, but can be applied to those with intellectual disabilities, where appropriate. In the UK, ICD-10 is most commonly used to classify mental disorders.

Types of psychotic disorders (as defined in ICD-10 [2]) include:

- Schizophrenia (this can be subdivided into paranoid, hebephrenic, catatonic or simple schizophrenia)

- Delusional disorder

- Acute and transient psychotic disorders

- Induced delusional disorder

- Schizoaffective disorder.

Psychotic symptoms can also be seen in severe mood disorders (e.g. bipolar affective disorder, depression or mania). In these cases, the symptoms are often mood congruent (e.g. grandiose delusions in a manic episode) (see Table 6.1).

In adults with moderate to severe/profound intellectual disabilities, it may be more difficult to elicit all the symptoms required for a diagnosis using ICD-10 or DSM-IV. Psychosis is therefore more likely to be defined in broader terms than that of the general population.

A DSM-IV [3] diagnosis of schizophrenia differs somewhat when compared to ICD-10, as it requires a month's history of characteristic symptoms (or shorter, if treatment commenced within this time), as well as some continuous signs of the disorder for at least six months (which can include prodromal or residual symptoms). It also requires a reduction in social or occupational functioning, when compared to premorbid levels. DSM-IV classifies hebephrenic schizophrenia as disorganized schizophrenia.

DSM-IV also specifies that where there is a history of autism or another pervasive developmental disorder, a diagnosis of schizophrenia can be made only if there are prominent delusions or hallucinations present for at least one month (or shorter if treatment commenced within this time).

The Diagnostic Criteria for Psychiatric Disorders for use with adults with Learning Disabilities/Mental Retardation (DC-LD) [4] is a classification system that has been

Table 6.1 Summary of ICD-10 criteria for schizophrenia [2]

At least one of A or at least two of B present for most of the time for at least one month:

A:

- Thought echo, thought insertion or withdrawal or thought broadcasting.
- Delusions of control, influence or passivity, referred to body or limb movements or specific thoughts, actions or sensations or delusional perception.
- Hallucinatory voices giving a running commentary or discussing the patient between themselves, or hallucinatory voices coming from some part of the body.
- Persistent delusions that are culturally inappropriate and completely impossible.

B:

- Persistent hallucinations in any modality, when accompanied by delusions or persistent overvalued ideas.
- Breaks or interpolations in the train of thought, leading to incoherence or irrelevant speech, or neologisms.
- Catatonic behaviour.
- Negative symptoms.

Schizophrenia can be categorized further into paranoid, hebephrenic or catatonic schizophrenia.

designed to work alongside ICD-10 in order to provide an operationalized framework for making a psychiatric diagnosis in people with moderate to severe/profound intellectual disabilities.

Definitions within non-affective psychotic disorders in DC-LD [4] include:

- Schizophrenic/delusional episode or disorder

- Schizoaffective episode or disorder

- Other non-affective psychotic disorders.
  Table 6.2 shows the DC-LD criteria for schizophrenia.

6.3 Epidemiology

The prevalence of schizophrenia in the general population is around 1%. There is an ongoing debate as to what the prevalence of schizophrenia is in people with intellectual disabilities; several studies report prevalence as 3% [1].

Table 6.2 Summary of DC-LD criteria for schizophrenic/delusional episode [4]

A: The symptoms/signs are not a direct consequence of any other psychiatric or physical disorder or a result of prescribed or illegal drugs or alcohol.

B: The criteria for schizoaffective episode are not met. (In DC–LD – unlike ICD–10 – a diagnosis of schizoaffective disorder trumps a diagnosis of schizophrenic/delusional episode).

C: One of item groups 1, 2 or 3 are met:

    1. One of the following symptoms present on most days for at least two weeks:

        a. Third-person auditory hallucinations discussing the person amongst themselves.

        b. Hallucinatory voices coming from some part of the body.

        c. Impossible/fantastic delusions (delusions which are culturally inappropriate and completely impossible).

        d. Thought insertion or withdrawal or broadcasting, or thought echo or delusions of control, influence or passivity, or delusional perception or hallucinatory voices giving a running commentary.

    2. One of the following present for most of the time during one month, or some time every day for at least a month:

        a. Delusions which are not mood congruent.

        b. Hallucinations (in any sensory modality) which are not mood congruent.

    3. Two of the following present on most days for at least two weeks:

        a. Delusions which are not mood congruent.

        b. Hallucinations which are not mood congruent.

        c. Catatonic symptoms.

        d. Negative symptoms, where there is definite evidence that this is a change from the individual's premorbid state.

        e. Disordered form of thought, where there is definite evidence that this is a change from the individual's premorbid state.

A recent population study has found that the standardized incidence ratio for first-episode psychosis in adults with learning disability is 10.0 (95% confidence interval 2.1−29.3), when compared to the general population [5].

Point prevalence rates of clinical diagnosis of psychotic disorder (including schizoaffective disorder) have been found to be 5.8% in adults with mild intellectual disabilities and 3.5% in those with moderate to profound intellectual disabilities [6]. This difference may, however, be a reflection of the difficulty in diagnosing people with more severe intellectual disabilities with a psychotic illness, rather than a true reflection of prevalence rates (see Chapter 2 on communication).

6.4 Aetiology and risk factors

It is helpful to think of aetiology by considering biological, psychological and social factors. When considering particular triggers to illness for an individual, it can also be helpful to think of aetiology using a predisposing, precipitating and perpetuating framework. Aetiology is likely to be multifactorial.

Much of the information on risk factors is extrapolated from data collected from people without intellectual disabilities. Several risk factors predispose to both intellectual disabilities and psychosis and it is not clear how much a low IQ itself is a risk factor for psychosis and how much of this is due to common risk factors.

Table 6.3 summarises the aetiological factors of psychotic disorders

Table 6.3   Aetiology and risk factors: possible biological, psychological and social factors

Biological factors:

- **Genetics:** A number of genes have been identified which are felt to be linked to a predisposition to psychosis: this is likely to be polygenic. Further research into this area is ongoing.

- **Neurochemistry:** Historically, dopamine overactivity was felt to be related to psychosis. It is now acknowledged that the neurochemistry behind this is more complex and is likely to involve a number of neurotransmitters, including dopamine and serotonin.

- **Neuroanatomy:** Small hippocampi and large ventricles are some of the radiological features identified in people with schizophrenia.

- Pregnancy and birth complications may be important in the aetiology of schizophrenia in people with intellectual disabilities [7].

- Cannabis use is known to increase the risk of psychosis [8].

Psychological factors:

- **IQ:** Low IQ itself has been found to be a risk factor for schizophrenia in a population-based study of 18-year-old males conscripted into the Swedish army. This may be a direct result of cognitive impairment (e.g. leading to false beliefs and perceptions), or there may be a common risk factor that links both low IQ and psychosis, such as abnormal brain development [9].

- Cognitive difficulties may result in delusions or disordered thinking.

Social factors:

- **Life events:** One study has identified that a single exposure to life events is significantly associated with schizophrenia in people with intellectual disabilities [10].

- Poor social network.

- Poor help seeking behaviours.

6.5 Clinical features and diagnosis

As mentioned previously, there are a number of disorders that present with features of psychosis. Common types of psychotic disorders (as categorized in ICD-10) are summarized below: [2]

- **Schizophrenia:** A chronic psychotic illness that can be either continuous or episodic. Episodes can be followed by periods of partial or complete remission. In some cases of schizophrenia, specific cognitive deficits and a functional decline can be seen which should not be confused with a diagnosis of intellectual disability itself, which is present from an early age. Schizophrenia can be further categorized as follows:

  - **Paranoid schizophrenia:** Features are predominantly that of paranoid delusions, and auditory hallucinations.

  - **Hebephrenic schizophrenia:** Affective changes are noted: either flattened, shallow, incongruous or inappropriate affect. Aimless or disjointed behaviours may be seen. Delusions and hallucinations are less evident.

  - **Catatonic schizophrenia:** Catatonic symptoms include excitement, posturing, negativism, waxy flexibility, rigidity, stupor and command automatisms.

- **Delusional disorder:** A disorder characterized by one, or a number of related delusions, which do not meet the criteria for schizophrenia. Symptoms of schizophrenia (e.g. passivity phenomena and thought insertion, withdrawal and broadcast) are not seen.

- **Acute and transient psychotic disorder:** A short-lived episode of psychosis, which can be triggered by social stressors, and resolves completely within a short period of time.

- **Induced delusional disorder:** A delusional disorder in which an individual develops a delusion that is shared with a close associate. The belief was not held before contact with the other person and often resolves following geographical separation. This is commonly known as folie à deux. Individuals who are more suggestible are more likely to have an induced delusional disorder.

- **Schizoaffective disorder:** A disorder that has prominent features of both schizophrenia and an affective disorder (either depression or mania, or both), with neither the psychotic or affective symptoms predominating. This may often have an episodic pattern.

Clinical features of schizophrenia

Clinical features of schizophrenia can be divided into positive and negative symptoms.

Positive symptoms

- **Delusions:** A fixed, unshakeable belief that is false or culturally inappropriate. Delusions can be paranoid (which can include grandiose or persecutory delusions), bizarre or impossible. Adults with intellectual disabilities can sometimes be 'talked out' of delusional beliefs. However, they may repeat the belief and continue to talk about it on a number of occasions [4].

- **Hallucinations:** These are often auditory hallucinations (e.g. an abnormal perception in an auditory modality – sound or voice). Hallucinations that are found in schizophrenia can include hearing voices providing a running commentary or third-person auditory hallucinations. Command hallucinations may also be present. In adults with intellectual disabilities, the extent of degree of hallucination will be dependent on the adult's language ability. It may be difficult for an individual to report symptoms, but they may be seen to be talking to themselves or responding in some other way to internal perceptions (e.g. looking round the room, as if something was there).

- **Abnormalities of thought:** This can include thought disorder, thought insertion, thought withdrawal and thought broadcast.

- **Passivity phenomena:** This can include made thoughts, made actions and made emotions.

Negative symptoms

- Apathy

- Poverty of speech

- Blunting of emotions.

Adults with intellectual disabilities may present with additional symptoms, as suggested in DC-LD [4] such as:

- Abnormal or challenging behaviour

- Appearing frightened, worried or perplexed

- Appearing to be talking to themselves or behaving as if there is someone else in the room

- May be 'talked out' of delusion, but will repeat belief soon after

- Tendency to social withdrawal or isolation.

Case vignette 6.1

Mr M is a 25-year-old gentleman with mild intellectual disability, who lives at home with his family. He attends day centres three days a week. He has some verbal skills and uses short phrases to communicate.

His parents and day centre staff report a three-month history of increasing isolation and social withdrawal. He has been reluctant to go to the day centre over the past month.

Over the past two weeks his family have noticed that he has become increasingly preoccupied with the television and he has started to express a belief that the television is communicating with him. He has recently started to think that the radio is also communicating with him. He has been seen to be talking to himself at times, although he denies this, and on occasion he has stood up and walked out of the living room, for no reason. This is out of character for him.

Difficulties in making a diagnosis of psychosis

In adults with intellectual disabilities, psychotic illness may present with atypical features, making identification of the illness and subsequent diagnosis challenging.

Adults with good verbal communication are likely to be able to describe symptoms such as auditory hallucinations, passivity symptoms and thought insertion, withdrawal and broadcast. These symptoms may become more difficult to assess in adults with more limited verbal communication, and diagnosis will require a greater focus on observation and collateral history. Therefore, there may be a group of people with psychosis and severe/profound intellectual disabilities who remain undiagnosed and possibly untreated.

Diagnostic overshadowing is a term used when an individual's behaviours are attributed to their intellectual disability, thereby missing other causes of mental illness (see also Chapters 2 and 3).

Care must be taken to carefully consider whether there could be any underlying cause for a change in behaviour. This highlights the importance of having a high degree of suspicion and conducting a detailed assessment when considering a diagnosis of psychosis in an adult with intellectual disability.

Case vignette 6.2

Miss C is a 34-year-old woman with moderate learning disabilities who attends a day centre and has some verbal communication skills up to three-word sentences. She is reported to be distracted, muttering to herself and becoming aggressive towards staff and other service users.

This carried on for several weeks before a referral to the community learning disabilities team was made. Staff at the day centre and her home carers considered that her change in behaviour was related to her learning disabilities rather than a change in her mental state. By the time of assessment, she had become increasingly restless, unable to settle at night and she was not able to link her words together to make sense. The assessing psychiatrist made a diagnosis of psychosis.

6.6 Differential diagnosis

As mentioned previously, it can be difficult to make a diagnosis of psychotic illness in an adult with intellectual disability. Although there is a risk of under-diagnosing psychotic illness, due to the nature of the presentation, it is also important to be aware of a number of other diagnoses that may present with similar symptoms to psychosis.

Some differential diagnoses to consider:

- Physical illness – including:

  - Epilepsy – in particular, temporal lobe epilepsy

  - Intracerebral conditions (e.g. space occupying lesion)

  - Infection (e.g. urinary or respiratory tract infection, meningitis)

  - Endocrine causes (e.g. hyper/hypothyroidism)

- Hearing or visual impairment (e.g. hallucinations or illusions due to visual impairment can be seen in Charles Bonnet syndrome)

- Causes of pain or distress (e.g. toothache, earache, constipation or menstrual pain).

• Drug or alcohol-related causes – including:

- Delirium tremens

- Alcoholic hallucinosis

- Drug induced psychosis

- Sensitivity to prescribed medication.

• Other psychiatric illness – including:

- Affective illness

- Anxiety disorder

- Post-traumatic stress disorder (PTSD).

• Dementia – (e.g. visual hallucinations in Lewy-body dementia)

• ASD [11]

• Other differential diagnoses – sometimes challenging behaviour, or intellectual disability itself can be misdiagnosed as psychosis.

6.7 Assessment and investigations

Assessment should always take into account an individual's developmental level and consider including:

• History from patient (if applicable)

• Mental state examination, including observation of patient in different settings, if appropriate

- Thorough collateral history – ideally from a number of different people involved in patient's care

- Assessment of drug and alcohol use

- Risk assessment (including intentional and non-intentional risk to self and others and risk from others)

- Physical examination and investigations.

  A list of relevant physical investigations may include:

- Thorough physical examination, including assessment of BP, pulse and temperature

- Blood tests – including FBC, U&E, Ca, LFTs, CRP, ESR and TFTs

- Septic screen, if indicated (including MSU, Sputum culture, CXR)

- CT/MRI head and EEG if indicated and no contraindications. This may be difficult for some patients to tolerate and an assessment of the benefits and risks of the investigation will be required.

There are a number of useful checklists that can be used to identify psychiatric disorders in people with intellectual disabilities. These include: the Reiss screen, [12] the Mini PAS-ADDs (Mini Psychiatric Assessment Schedules for Adults with Developmental Disabilities), [13] the DASH-II (Diagnostic Assessment for the Severely Handicapped-II) [14] and the ADD (Assessment of Dual Diagnosis) [15]. These tools appear to be useful general indicators of psychiatric disorders, but are less helpful in determining the nature of the illness [16].

If used, they should be completed alongside a thorough clinical assessment.

6.8 Management

There is little research evidence on the treatment of psychotic disorders in adults with intellectual disabilities, and much of the rationale for treatment is extrapolated from research in the general population and from clinical experience.

Management is similar to management in those without intellectual disabilities, and can be considered using a biopsychosocial approach. Treatment should be tailored to the individual's needs. In the acute phase of the illness, management is likely to focus on accessing appropriate services, adequate risk assessment and ensuring the safety of the patient and others, as well as consideration and initiation of medication. After resolution of the acute phase of the illness, management is more likely to focus on insight-related work and relapse prevention planning.

Individuals with intellectual disabilities have the right to access the same health services (including mental health services) as those without intellectual disabilities, as stated in the government paper, *Valuing People, 2001* [17]. Services in the UK form a network of primary and secondary care that comprises general practitioners, accident and emergency departments and learning disability teams. Additional resources may be provided by crisis intervention teams, assertive outreach teams and early intervention in psychosis teams. Adults with intellectual disabilities and a diagnosis of psychosis or other severe and enduring mental illness may be followed up under the care programme approach (CPA).

A thorough risk assessment, identifying any intentional and unintentional risks to the patient from themselves and others (including self-neglect), as well as any risks to others, will help identify where a person can be managed.

Wherever an individual is supported, it is important to consider biological, psychological and social interventions:

Biological

Antipsychotics are the main type of medication used in the treatment of psychosis; they can be categorized into typical and atypical antipsychotic medications. Typical antipsychotics include haloperidol, chlorpromazine and flupentixol. A number of typical antipsychotics are available as a depot preparation. Typical antipsychotics are associated with extrapyramidal side effects (EPSEs), which include acute dystonias, parkinsonism, akathisia and tardive dyskinesia (see also Chapter 14).

Atypical antipsychotics are not as strongly associated with EPSEs. They include risperidone, olanzapine and clozapine. Risperidone is available in a depot preparation. Side effects in this group can include weight gain and hyperglycaemia.

Antipsychotics are often associated with sedation and a number of antipsychotics can lower the seizure threshold. Careful consideration of medication type, balancing the individual's needs with the treatment and side effect profile of the medication is required, particularly if the patient has a history of epilepsy or significant physical health problems. Regular physical health checks (including cardiovascular and endocrine review) should be conducted. The National Institute for Clinical Excellence (NICE) guidelines for schizophrenia (update) [18] suggest that people with schizophrenia have a physical health review by their GP at least once a year (see Table 6.4). Results should be communicated to the care coordinator or responsible psychiatrist.

Table 6.4   (amended) NICE guidelines for schizophrenia – update (2009) – summary of recommendations for initiating antipsychotics in schizophrenia [18 – amended]

- In newly diagnosed schizophrenia, oral antipsychotic medication should be offered.
- The choice of antipsychotic should be made by the service user and healthcare professional, after discussion of benefits and side effect profile (including extrapyramidal side effects, metabolic side effects and other side effects).
- The carer's views (where the service user agrees) should also be considered in the choice of antipsychotic.
- More than one antipsychotic should not be used at any one time (except for short periods of time, for example when changing medication).
- If an individual has not responded adequately to treatment, despite sequential trials of two different antipsychotics (including one which is a non-clozapine, second generation antipsychotic), clozapine should be offered.

An ECG prior to starting antipsychotics and at regular intervals thereafter is useful to monitor any ECG abnormalities, in particular any QT prolongation. The NICE guidelines for schizophrenia (update) [18] suggest that an ECG is offered before starting antipsychotics if there is any evidence of cardiovascular risk factors (including past history), the person is being admitted as an inpatient, or if an ECG is specified on the summary of product characteristics (SPCs) of the antipsychotic.

Neuroleptic malignant syndrome is a rare side effect of some antipsychotic medications. It is characterized by an altered consciousness state, muscle rigidity, hyperthermia and autonomic dysfunction (including labile blood pressure and sweating). Antipsychotic medication should be stopped and urgent medical attention is required, as it is a potentially fatal condition.

Small studies in the literature show that clozapine appears to be efficacious and safe in people with intellectual disabilities; [19, 20] however, careful monitoring of side effects is recommended [20].

A Cochrane review in 2004 did not find any sufficiently detailed randomized controlled trials that examined antipsychotic medication versus placebo for people with both schizophrenia and intellectual disabilities. They highlighted the need for further research in this area [21]. See also Chapter 14.

Psychological

A number of psychological interventions can be of benefit in adults without intellectual disabilities. There is not yet detailed research into how effective these may be in adults with intellectual disabilities. Amongst other things, psychological approaches can focus on coping with psychotic symptoms, insight-related work and relapse prevention planning. Obviously any psychological therapy must be tailored to the individual's developmental level.

Psychological approaches that may be considered:

- Cognitive behavioural therapy

- Family and carer interventions

- Psycho-educational groups may be beneficial in improving patient understanding of psychosis [22].

Psychological therapies are discussed further in Chapter 15.

Social

Practical social interventions, tailored to an individual's needs, are important in order to support both the patient and their support network. These can include:

- Person centred plan.

- Comprehensive needs assessment by care managers (if not previously known to care management) – including consideration of accommodation, daytime activities and social support.

- Community care review by care managers (if known to care management) if there is a change in the individual's needs.

- Carer's assessment to identify problems associated with the caring role if the person resides with his/her family.

Case vignette 6.3

Mr S, who has mild learning disabilities, was diagnosed as suffering with paranoid schizophrenia. He was initially admitted to hospital where he made good progress on antipsychotic medication. Whilst on the ward he was also placed on a self-medication regime monitored by the nursing staff and the pharmacist. He completed the programme successfully and became involved in occupational therapy and ward-based groups.

On discharge, he was placed on CPA. He was referred to nursing for support around taking his medication and in order to monitor any side effects. He was referred to speech and language therapy in order to help him communicate his worries about 'wires coming out of the walls' and was referred to a local voluntary organization who run drop-in groups for adults with mental illness and persistent psychotic symptoms.

6.9 Outcome/prognosis

As with the challenge of diagnosis in people with psychosis and intellectual disabilities, it is equally difficult measuring outcomes. This can make it difficult to examine prognosis.

One study observed that people with schizophrenia-spectrum psychoses and intellectual disabilities have more observable psychopathology and negative symptoms when compared to a group without intellectual disabilities [23]. Another study in youths referred with early onset psychosis and intellectual disabilities found that patients with psychosis not otherwise specified and moderate or severe intellectual disabilities had a poorer outcome [24].

6.10 Genetic syndromes and psychosis

22q11 deletion syndrome (also known as velo-cardio-facial syndrome or DiGeorge syndrome) is a syndrome resulting from a microdeletion at the q11.2 band of chromosome 22 [25]. Features include somatic abnormalities such cleft palate and congenital heart defects and mild to moderate intellectual disabilities. It is strongly associated with an increased risk of psychosis – schizophrenia has been shown to develop in around 24% of cases [26]. Other features can include facial characteristics.

Prader Willi syndrome (PWS) results from a small deletion on the paternal chromosome 15 (60–70% of cases), whilst about 25% of cases are caused by inheriting two chromosome 15s from the mother (maternal disomy). A few cases result from a translocation or an imprinting error involving chromosome 15. Its main features are hypotonia, hypogonadism, obesity and central nervous system and endocrine gland dysfunction which causes varying degrees of intellectual disabilities and emotional disorders (http://pwsa.co.uk/main.php). Recent research has revealed that the sub-type of PWS due to maternal disomy is associated with high rates of psychiatric illness, typically presenting as affective psychosis [27].

References

1. Smiley, E. (2005) Epidemiology of mental health problems in adults with learning disability: an update. *Advances in Psychiatric Treatment*, **11**, 214–222.

2. World Health Organization (1992) The ICD-10 Classification of Mental and Behavioural Disorders: Clinical Descriptions and Diagnostic Guidelines, Chapter V: Mental and Behavioural Disorders, World Health Organization, Geneva.

3. American Psychiatric Association (2000) Diagnostic and Statistical Manual of Mental Disorders, 4th edn, (DSM-IV), American Psychiatric Publishing, Washington, DC.

4. Royal College of Psychiatrists (2001) DC-LD: Diagnostic Criteria for Psychiatric Disorders for use with Adults with Learning Disabilities/Mental Retardation, Gaskell Press, London.

5. Cooper, S.A., Smiley, E., Morrison, J. et al. (2007) Psychosis and adults with intellectual disabilities. Prevalence, incidence and related factors. Social Psychiatry and Psychiatric Epidemiology, 42, 530–536.

6. Cooper, S.A., Smiley, E., Morrison, J. et al. (2007) Mental ill health in adults with intellectual disabilities: prevalence and associated factors. British Journal of Psychiatry, 190, 27–35.

7. O'Dwyer, J.M. (1997) Schizophrenia in people with intellectual disability: the role of pregnancy and birth complications. Journal of Intellectual Disability Research, 41, 238–251.

8. Luzi, S., Morrison, P.D., Powell, J. et al. (2008) What is the mechanism whereby cannabis use increases risk of psychosis? Neurotoxicity Research, 14, 105–112.

9. David, A.S., Malmberg, A., Brandt, L. et al. (1997) IQ and risk for schizophrenia: a population-based cohort study. Psychological Medicine, 27, 1311–1323.

10. Tsakanikos, E., Bouras, N., Costello, H. et al. (2007) Multiple exposure to life events and clinical psychopathology in adults with intellectual disability. Social Psychiatry and Psychiatric Epidemiology, 42, 24–28.

11. Palucka, A.M., Bradley, E. and Lunsky, Y. (2008) A case of unrecognised Intellectual Disability and Autism misdiagnosed as Schizophrenia: are there lessons to be learned? Mental Health Aspects of Developmental Disabilities, 11, 55–60.

12. Reiss, S. (1988) Test Manual for the Reiss Screen for Maladaptive Behaviour, International Diagnostic Systems, Orlando Park.

13. Prosser, H., Moss, S., Costello, H. et al. (1997) The Mini PAS-ADD: An Assessment Schedule for the Detection of Mental Health Needs in Adults with Learning Disability (Mental Retardation), Hester Adrian Research Centre, University of Manchester, Manchester.

14. Matson, J.L. (1995) The Diagnostic Assessment for the Severely Handicapped-II, Scientific Publishers, Baton Rouge.

15. Matson, J.L. and Bamburg, J.W. (1998) Reliability of the assessment of dual diagnosis (ADD). Research in Developmental Disabilities, 19, 89–95.

16. Myrbakk, E. and von Tetzchner, S. (2008) Screening individuals with intellectual disability for psychiatric disorders: comparison of four measures. American Journal on Mental Retardation, 113 (1), 54–70.

17. Department of Health (2001) Valuing People: A New Strategy for Learning Disability for the 21st Century.

18. Department of Health (2009) Schizophrenia – Core Interventions in the Treatment and Management of Schizophrenia in Primary and Secondary Care (Update), National Institute for Clinical Excellence.

19. Antonacci, D.J. and de Groot, C.M. (2000) Clozapine treatment in a population of adults with mental retardation. The Journal of Clinical Psychiatry, 61, 22–25.

20. Thalayasingam, S., Alexander, R.T. and Singh, I. (2004) The use of clozapine in adults with intellectual disability. Journal of Intellectual Disability Research, 48, 572–579.

21. Duggan, L. and Brylewski, J. (2004) Antipsychotic medication versus placebo for people with both schizophrenia and learning disability. *Cochrane Database of Systematic Reviews* 4 (Art. No.: CD000030).

22. Crowley, V., Rose, J., Smith, J. *et al.* (2008) Psycho-educational groups for people with a dual diagnosis of psychosis and mild intellectual disability: a preliminary study. *Journal of Intellectual Disabilities*, **2**, 25–39.

23. Bouras, N., Martin, G., Leese, M. *et al.* (2004) Schizophrenia-spectrum psychoses in people with and without intellectual disability. *Journal of Intellectual Disability Research*, **48**, 548–555.

24. Friedlander, R.I. and Donnelly, T. (2004) Early-onset psychosis in youth with intellectual disability. *Journal of Intellectual Disability Research*, **48**, 540–547.

25. Shprintzen, R.J. (2008) Velo-cardio-facial syndrome: 30 years of study. *Developmental Disabilities Research Reviews*, **14**, 3–10.

26. Murphy, K.C., Jones, L.A. and Owen, M.J. (1999) High rates of schizophrenia in adults with velo-cardio-facial syndrome. *Archives of General Psychiatry*, **56**, 940–945.

27. Soni, S., Whittington, J., Holland, A.J. *et al.* (2008) The phenomenology and diagnosis of psychiatric illness in people with Prader – Willi syndrome. *Psychological Medicine*, **38**, 1505–1514.

Further reading

www.intellectualdisability.info.

7 Mental Health Aspects of Autism Spectrum Disorders*

Peter Carpenter
Kingswood CLDT, Bristol, UK

7.1 Introduction

Autism spectrum disorder (ASD) is the collective term currently used for people with ICD-10-defined childhood autism, Asperger's syndrome or atypical autism (see Box 7.1). In the last few years there has been an increasing emphasis on the social and communicative impairments necessary in order to make a diagnosis which are thought of as an impairment relative to the person's cognitive and practical abilities, rather than as an absolute level of ability or skill. As a result, an increasing number of more socially able and integrated individuals are being recognized as having a relative impairment of social interaction and communication and thus being diagnosed with the condition. It is now recognized that most people with ASD are of normal or high intelligence (as measured using an IQ test).

7.2 Causes of ASD

The cause of ASD is unknown but best considered to be a multifactorial disease. The distribution of ASD within families indicates that it cannot be caused by a single gene but must involve the interaction of several. Most individuals with ASD have a family history of ASD or learning difficulties such as dyslexia. Some individuals

* The current terminology used by the UK government is autistic spectrum conditions.

Intellectual Disability Psychiatry: a practical handbook   Angela Hassiotis, Diana Andrea Barron and Ian Hall (eds)
© 2009 John Wiley & Sons, Ltd

without a family history of ASD have a personal history of prenatal or infantile neurological insult such as encephalitis.

Assessments of the skills and impairments of people with ASD generally show a problem with neurones communicating between areas of the brain, with a wide variety of patterns of deficits reported. This appears to cause a variety of processing difficulties, but with some islets of ability and processing strengths. The overall outcome appears to be the impairment of social and verbal interactions, combined with a retreat into ritual and routine [1].

Box 7.1   ICD-10 Criteria for the autism spectrum disorders

These are the anomalies specified in the diagnostic guidelines for ICD-10 diagnosis, given under each area of impairment.

Unlike DSM IV, the ICD-10 guidelines do not specify the number of anomalies required in each domain for that person to qualify as having difficulties in that domain; it is left to clinical judgement.

- Qualitative impairments in reciprocal social interaction:

  - Lack of responses to other people's emotions

  - Lack of modulation of behaviour according to social context

  - Poor use of social signals

  - Poor use of non-verbal signals to regulate social interactions

  - Weak integration of social, emotional and communicative behaviours

  - Lack of socio-emotional reciprocity

  - Failure to develop peer relationships involving mutual sharing.

- Qualitative impairment in communication:

  - Delay in development of language (without attempts to use other methods of communication)

  - Lack of social usage of language skills

  - Repetitive speech

- Poor synchrony and reciprocity in conversational interchange

- Lack of emotional response to other people's verbal and non-verbal overtures.

- Poor flexibility in language expression

- Impaired use of cadence or emphasis to modulate communication

- Impaired use of gesture to augment spoken communication

- Impairment in make-believe and social imitative play

- Relative lack of creativity and fantasy in thought processes

• Restricted, repetitive and stereotyped patterns of behaviour:

- Tendency to impose rigidity and routine on day-to-day living

- Resistance to change in environment or routines

- Attachment to unusual objects, or interests.

- Non-functional routines

- Interest in non-functional elements of objects

- Motor stereotypies.

If meet the above and onset before age 3 = childhood autism F84.0
If only meet two of criteria or onset after age 3 = atypical autism F84.1
If no delay in development of communication or cognitive development (may or may not have impaired communication) = Asperger's syndrome F84.5

7.3 How to make a diagnosis of mental illness in ASD

People with ASD have many of the same emotional needs as other people. They often report being lonely and wanting a close friend, though they may not have the skills to acquire one. Having an ASD does not determine one's precise personality or additional mental disorder. Many people with ASD, especially the milder forms, are highly successful in business.

People with ASD have similar times of crisis to other people in their lives though some may seem more catastrophic. Children with ASD have often created niches for themselves at home and school through their adolescence, and the abrupt and total change that comes with leaving school can produce a dramatic regression or anxiety state. So can other major transitions such as loss of carers (usually parents) or change of home.

The biggest problem in diagnosing mental disorder in people with autism must be with those who have limited communication and cannot describe what they want or are doing or feeling. However, communication is a spectrum both of ability to use words, and of interest in communicating with others (further information on communications can be found in Chapter 2) (see Box 7.2 for issues specific to ASD).

Box 7.2   Problems with communication specific to individuals with ASD

- May not be able to talk at all and not have learned other forms of communication.

- May repeat phrases they have heard (either immediate repetition, as in echolalia, or at a later time, often called 'tape recorder speech') but with no understanding of what the words mean.

- May be using brief, 'telegram style' speech.

- May speak but not recognize need to tell person about problem.

- May not have vocabulary to describe problem.

7.4 Assessment

In order to carry out an assessment of mental illness in a person with ASD it is important to have prior information available usually from paid or family carers who are familiar with the person's behaviour over time and who can lead in guiding how best to interact with the person. The person should be seen in a comfortable setting; otherwise a low stimulus environment should be chosen with as few people in the room as possible [2].

The approach to examination where there is lack of verbal communication should be to observe for interests, repetitions, avoidances. The clinician should reflect repetitions back and watch the response. In addition, one may tentatively try to interrupt repetitive behaviour, or touch the person to look at the response. The instructions or questions must be short and put in simple language and sufficient time should be allowed for a response. Ask for facts first (e.g. What time do you go to bed?). Direct questions should be followed by a request for the person to give examples.

Particular issues to be considered during the assessment of a person with ASD are summarized in Box 7.3 and occur in several domains.

Box 7.3   Problems in diagnosing mental disorder in ASD

Reporting
May not occur to person to tell someone about how they feel.

Assessment
- Facial expression/body language may not reflect emotion the person is feeling (e.g. may be very 'flat' all the time or smile all the time).

- Vocal intonation may not reflect emotion the person is feeling (e.g. may sound flat and be thought to be angry, when this is normal intonation style).

- May not be able to use correct vocabulary to describe emotion, or abstract feeling (e.g. that 'depressed', or that have 'butterflies in the stomach').

- May respond to questions concretely and literally and be misunderstood (e.g. Do you hear voices? – Yes – I hear you now).

- May not process long sentences correctly, so pick out key words, guess what was said and reply or do accordingly (classically, do what told *not* to do, as did not register the 'not').

- Sensory or processing overload may produce bizarre escape behaviour.

- Features of regression may dominate and mask causative presentation.

Interpretation
- Concrete explanations may seem bizarre and psychotic.

- Phenomena may reflect a lower emotional developmental stage. For example, imaginary friend, magical thinking in adult.

- Boundary between fixed, repetitive ideas may merge into delusions.

- Imaginary world used to model real world (or to entertain self) may appear to be a delusion.

7.5 Challenging behaviour in ASD

A high proportion of people with difficult challenging behaviour (see Chapter 9) have an ASD.

Often, challenging behaviour in autism occurs because the carers do not recognize the person's sensitivities or desires and may make assumptions that the person will want to take part in the same things that the carer wants to do.

Case vignette 7.1

A young man with autism is being restrained several times a day; it takes four people to do so safely and four stay in the room with him at all times. He does little but is 'entertained' by the television being on all day, which staff watch and chat about.

His behaviour dramatically improves when the television is turned off, and three of the four staff sit outside of the room with only one person in the room who plays with him, with sensory toys interspersed by physical activity.

7.6 Comorbid disorders in ASD

Anxiety-related disorders

Anxiety is common in autism and probably more so than in the general population. It can lead to all the common signs of distress but also may trigger a range of anxiety-related disorders.

Sleep disorders in autism may be related to attention deficit hyperactivity disorder (ADHD) or underlying brain disorders, but are most commonly related to anxiety. They can often be improved by bedtime routines that are relaxing. Pharmacological intervention may be needed, and melatonin has become fashionable within autism. However, one should be cautious of long-term use of any hypnotic.

Often, due to the 'one shot learning' style of memory, one unpleasant experience may lead to avoidance and a phobic reaction. A common phobia, for example is of dogs.

More able people with ASDs are aware that they are different and can be keen to pass as normal. They can develop a severe social performance anxiety and phobia.

People with ASD classically have repetitive rituals and routines. In general, these are usually done for pleasure, to calm down or to reduce or block out the stress in the world. In some, though, anxiety develops into obsessions and compulsions. This can be something simple like insisting all windows are closed, or flushing four times, but can also be more classical obsessions such as avoiding touching things in case one hurts others by contamination, or over-washing, checking repetitively, or insisting things are returned to the same place by reversing the movement by which they left their position.

Features that may help a clinician decide a repetitive activity is an obsession rather than a ritual are:

- Does the person seem anxious at time of repetitive behaviour?

- Does the person show signs of pleasure around activity?

- Is the person angry or anxious if interrupted?

- How far does the activity dominate his/her life?

Obsessions tend to dominates the person's life and, when interrupted, they cause anxiety rather than anger.

Given the importance of anxiety in powering this disorder, selective serotonin reuptake inhibitors (SSRIs) and related anxiolytics can help the person cope with external control of the obsession and any related depression (see Chapter 14).

Environmental adaptation can also help reduce anxiety more generally and thus also reduce the intensity of the obsession. In addition, those with verbal skills may be able to use cognitive behaviour treatment (CBT). The danger of CBT is that the self-examination required may become a preoccupation in its own right.

Case vignette 7.2

A man with Asperger's syndrome lives at home with his parents. He will not touch his parents and will not touch door handles or fomites without covering his hand with his sleeve. He washes for one hour in the shower each day using enormous quantities of shower gel. Assessment reveals he is frightened of harming his parents by giving them germs. He is treated with a combination of antidepressants, education on germs and the immune system, by education on anxiety and the anxiety response and by goal setting in touching, response prevention and in reducing his washing. He moves to his own flat where he copes well with reasonable levels of self-washing though this increases at times of stress.

ADHD

ADHD can exist as an additional diagnosis in ASD, though casual reading of ICD-10 may make one feel that a diagnosis of ASD makes it impossible to also diagnose ADHD. Many people with ASD have no problems with restlessness or distractibility. Some individuals quickly get bored and entertain themselves by irritating others for a dramatic response.

The problem is deciding whether the level of restlessness or distractibility is in keeping with the person's general level of functioning, or more severe than one would expect. If it is more severe then it probably needs treating and stimulant medication may be considered in addition to behavioural programmes. Stimulant medication can be very effective in slowing a person down and making them feel calmer and more focussed. However, stimulants may carry an increased risk in autism of provoking seizures and tics [3].

Mood disorders

People with autism can suffer two types of mood disorder (see Chapter 5). The first is a general unstable mood that is rapidly changing, dependent on any recent event. This seems to be linked to a general lack of inner self-awareness, and be associated with a lack of emotional regulation. Management is difficult but mainly psychological with encouragement of maturation and self-awareness. Chemical mood stabilizers such as sodium valproate can sometimes help (see Chapter 14).

The second is major affective disorder. There is an association of a family history of affective disorder with ASD and severe depression and mania are probably the most common psychiatric disorders associated with ASD. It is important to make a distinction between the fleeting interests of a person in a manic phase and an intensity of interests found in individual with ASD.

Case vignette 7.3

A man with no verbal communication and autism becomes violent. Careful enquiry reveals that he is more reluctant to do any activity and is hitting out when people encourage him. He has lost interest in many of his favourite activities. He is most irritable in the morning, is losing weight and is sleeping for long periods. He does not appear to be in pain. He is rocking more. His key worker left a month ago. He returns to his old self within a few weeks of being placed on antidepressants. Carers realize that staff changes need to be planned.

Hypomania and agitated depression can appear almost identical in a person with poor speech and ASD. The most common prominent difference is the degree of sexual activity, which is unusual in agitated depression, except for comfort masturbation.

The major mood disorders respond to conventional pharmacological treatments.

Case vignette 7.4

A man with autism and limited speech is having mood swings lasting several days; when he is 'down' he is incontinent, stays in bed, is non-verbal and resists all attempts to go out. When hypomanic he sleeps less, vocalises excessively and constantly wants to go out. There is no clear trigger to the swings. They reduce with a mood stabilizer.

Schizophreniform disorders

People with ASD can suffer the same psychoses as anyone else. They can suffer an *acute and transient psychotic disorder* at times of crises or stress overload. They can become paranoid about others, just as most people do if they do not fully understand what is going on around them. So a person with ASD can be suspicious that people are talking about him/her, or that cars flash their lights at him/her. Most of these can be treated with a person being with them to provide reassurance, or with anxiolytics (classically SSRIs) or *low* doses of an antipsychotic.

Psychosis can also happen as part of a mood disorder. There is probably an over-diagnosis of schizophrenia in people with ASD due to the confusion of odd ideas or strange hobbies and interests with delusional thoughts and psychotic thinking patterns. Common difficulties leading to a diagnosis of psychosis in a person with ASD are shown in Box 7.4.

Box 7.4   Symptoms of psychosis and ASD

- Consider reasons for strange behaviour other than schizophrenia.

- May fail to distinguish obsessional thoughts from external hallucinations.

- Imaginary friends or conjuring up of past friends may be misinterpreted as telepathy or 'being able to talk to friend over long distances'.

- Rigid or bizarre thinking may be confused with primary delusions.

- Tangential, overinclusive thinking may be confused with thought disorder.

A detailed history to explore the onset of the disorder and its presenting symptoms is of great importance. In general, however, the diagnosis is most likely to be made in individuals with substantial verbal skills who are able to describe their thoughts and experiences.

If it is decided that a person suffers with a psychotic illness, it is often worth starting the person on low dose antipsychotics first, to see how rapidly stress reduction reduces the symptoms. Most people with ASD respond well to conventional antipsychotic treatment.

Personality disorder

ASD is a neurodevelopmental disorder, affecting the processing of information. What personality the person develops as a result of this can vary and sometimes reach the severity of a personality disorder (PD). There is, however, a debate as to whether one should diagnose a personality disorder in people with ASD. It is not allowed to diagnose schizoid personality disorder in people with Asperger's syndrome, presumably as so many people with the syndrome are likely to meet this description. However some meet the criteria for dissocial PD, emotionally unstable PD or possibly paranoid PD.

Eating disorders

People with ASD have two types of eating disorder: pica and anorexia/bulimia. Pica generally occurs in the less able and is linked to developmental level, sensation seeking and lack of awareness of social propriety. Occasionally, it has been linked with lack of minerals such as iron deficiency.

Many of the more able people with ASD may have anorexia caused by a variety of things: an obsession, control of one's body, control of body shape, poor awareness of internal body sensations of hunger, naive ideas about body physiology or enjoyment of the reaction of others to the self-control. The degree of self-control can be phenomenal; maintaining lethally low weights, or, for example drinking and eating only at weekends. Conventional treatments that emphasize choice and responsibility are usually unsuccessful and the person may need education, SSRI antidepressants for anxiety and concrete target setting linked to external rewards.

People with ASD can also develop food fads; this may be due to sensory problems, such as only tolerating the most bland (or spicy) foods, or only tolerating lukewarm food. But it can also be due to habit formation or total imposition of the person's desires on others. It is very difficult to provide nutritiously appropriate food to a young man who only eats one brand of custard, and no other food. Carers often have to very slowly add other food stuffs in such small quantities that the person adapts and does not refuse all food. However this approach often needs the parents (and doctors) to be treated for anxiety as much as the person in question!

7.7 Sexual identity and paraphilias

Some adolescents with ASD develop sexual fetishes when they have a sexual pleasure associated with a specific experience.

People with ASD seem to like sex as much as anyone else (though sensitivity to touch may make mutual contact difficult). They also have difficulty with the skills needed to chat up other people. The effect of this combination is varied, particularly in those of normal intelligence. Some may depend on the internet for sexual stimulation and can become addicted to it.

When approaching others for sex, most find it easier to be chatted up than to chat up but lacking the social skills to extricate themselves from situations may lead to sexual abuse for both men and women with ASD.

As a result of poor identity and sexual experiences, there does seem to be a higher incidence of people with ASD wanting to change gender. This is often naive and can reflect an underlying confusion about sexual roles. Sexual education, social skills work and counselling is often helpful here.

The social peer of the same mental age as an adult with ASD is often a child. This does occasionally lead to sexual experimentation and more rarely to paedophilic predation.

Case vignette 7.5

A young man with Asperger's syndrome announces he wants to be a woman and cross-dresses. When assessed he talks about how women have a much easier time in society and everyone looks after them. Asked about sexual orientation he points out that he is not homosexual so when he changes gender he clearly will start to fancy men. Asked what he will do if he discovers that being a woman is not that nice, he responds that he will have his sex change reversed. A course of sexual education proves useful to him.

7.8 Substance misuse

People with ASD often learn that various substances are fun or helpful. Coffee (or sufficient water) may have a stimulating effect. Alcohol can help a person to become more sociable. Similarly, use of cannabis may introduce the user to an accepting and tolerant social group.

Alcohol abuse is relatively common in those with social anxiety. Cannabis use can become excessive and can trigger psychoses.

Motivational counselling with concrete targets is often needed. Environmental manipulation may reduce some of the stress that also drives the drinking (see Chapter 8).

7.9 Impulse disorders

A lot of people with autism appear to have much greater problems controlling impulses than one would expect from their other skills. This may simply be a feature of not learning many of the self-controls gained during social skill development. It may also be associated with mood disorder and distractability. It does, however, clearly lead to problems with many behaviours, including aggression. Some more able people with ASD have problems with socialized impulse disorders such as gambling. Gambling is designed to be psychologically compelling with the intermittent rewards and excitement of the gamble. It is very difficult to control in people with ASD when established and is best done with boundary setting and removing temptation.

Tourette's syndrome

Tourette's syndrome is said to be more common in ASD ([4], for a comprehensive review). It is important to distinguish the tics and verbal ejaculations of Tourette's syndrome from mannerisms, stereotypies or self-stimulation. Tourette tics stop during sleep in the same way as stereotypies. The treatment for Tourette's syndrome in ASD is little different from that in individuals without ASD and includes both psychological and pharmacological interventions.

Case vignette 7.6

A young man shouts out swear words and grunts when he gets tense with frustration. The shout is so loud he startles people about him. He has learnt at times to leave the room so he can grunt outside where no one hears him. He describes an inner tension before the grunt and shout that is discharged by the action. It is most obvious when he plays computer games and runs out of the room midway through them. He also has a facial tic. All improve with low dose risperidone.

Catatonia

Some people with ASD seem to have difficulty with movement; they can freeze when starting or in the middle of motion. This may happen suddenly in the middle of an activity such as eating, or be a difficulty moving through transitions such as visual barriers like doorways or colour changes in carpets. This difficulty often starts in adolescence and may need verbal prompts to break through, small physical prompts, or background rhythm such as music.

In a very few people this can escalate into full catatonic stupor. Once neuroleptic malignant syndrome and epilepsy have been excluded, the person should be treated conventionally with high dose lorazepam and electroconvulsive therapy [5].

Epilepsy

Epilepsy may be more common in ASD compared with others of similar ability. Abnormal rhythms can, however, show in EEGs of people with autism who do not clinically have epilepsy.

Diagnosis of partial seizures can be very difficult if the person has repetitive actions and refuses an EEG. For example a person who repetitively flickers their eyes may be self-stimulating or having a seizure or inducing a seizure.

Other disorders

Sensory integration disorders

Whilst the concept of sensory integration disorders is not included in the ICD-10 or DSM IV, there is widespread recognition that some people have difficulty with modulating or integrating their sensory experiences. This is common but not unique to autism [6] and may involve any of the senses: touch (receiving or using), hearing, vision, smell and taste but also vestibular senses and those of proprioception. There can be hyposensitivity, hypersensitivity or poor modulation which, for example, can be experienced as hypersensitivity to high pitched sound, making showers and echoing bathrooms painful; or as painful touch making being kissed politely or cuddled or restrained very painful. A lot of the more bizarre behaviours in people with autism can be explained by sensory anomalies.

Processing difficulties

A lot of people with ASD seem to have difficulty processing information on top of having sensory difficulties. They can be easily overloaded by a lot of things happening at once. This can make attending social or busy events very difficult and stressful and many become reluctant to leave their homes as a result.

This can also occur during conversation. Some people describe that they hear speech faster than they can process it. As the talker says more and more so the words jumble together and the person with ASD has to seize on words and guess what is being said. The result is that they often 'mishear' and may end up doing precisely what they were told *not* to do. The carer then interprets this as deliberate and gets annoyed, when it is in fact because the carer forgot to tell the person *what to do*, and to use short sentences, with uncomplicated phrasing.

Case vignette 7.7

A man with autism and no verbal skills constantly 'body pops', that is, moving his limbs, trunk and head. At one point it was feared he would damage his neck. He was observed to do it more when bored, and to have poor sense of joint position. His movements improved with weighted armbands to increase joint position feedback.

Case vignette 7.8

A man with autism and lack of verbal communication living in a flat suddenly becomes highly distressed. No cause can be found, until eventually the staff realize that the fire panel in the next door flat has a fault and is bleeping repetitively. The man quietens when the panel is repaired.

Case vignette 7.9

A man in hospital with a diagnosis of schizophrenia and Asperger's syndrome keeps his ears stuffed with tissue 'to keep the voices out'. Enquiry reveals he is sensitive to all noises, and is not hallucinating, but dampening his hearing. Ear mufflers prove more useful than antipsychotics for his symptoms.

ASDs are a complex group of disorders that can be further complicated by the presence of severe intellectual disabilities and other comorbidities, particularly challenging behaviour. Services, at least in parts of the UK, are under-resourced to deal with individuals with ASD and, frequently, specialist placements are found out of the individual's area of origin. The Department of Health (UK) announced a new epidemiological study to examine the prevalence, mental health and social care needs of adults with autism (2008) which will lead to the first ever strategy for adults with autism and related disorders.

References

1. Volkmar, F.R., Paul, R., Klin, A. and Cohen, D. (2005) *Handbook of Autism and Pervasive Developmental Disorders*, 3rd edn, 2 Vols, John Wiley & Sons, Inc., New Jersey.
2. Banks, R., Bush, A., Baker, P. *et al.* (2007) Challenging Behaviour: A Unified Approach, Royal College of Psychiatrists, British Psychological Society and Royal College of Speech and Language Therapists, London, CR 144. Available at: http://www.rcpsych.ac.uk/files/pdfversion/cr144.pdf.
3. Ghaziuddin, M. (2005) *Mental Health Aspects of Autism and Asperger Syndrome*, Jessica Kingsley Publishers, London and Philadelphia.
4. Robertson, M. (2000) Tourette syndrome, associated conditions and the complexities of treatment. *Brain*, **123**, 425–462.
5. Dhosshe D.M., Wing L., Ohta M. and Neumärker, K.-J. (eds) (2006) *Catatonia in Autism Spectrum Disorders*, International Review of Neurobiology, vol **72**, Academic Press, London.
6. Leekam, S.R., Neito, C., Libby, S.J. *et al.* (2006) Describing the sensory abnormalities of children and adults with autism. *Journal Autism Developmental Disorders*, **37**, 894–910.

Further reading

National Autistic Society at www.nas.org.uk.

Useful information on new initiatives and other resources may be found in the web site of the Department of Health http://www.dh.gov.uk.

8 Substance Misuse

Helen Miller and Emma Whicher
Adult Team National Deaf Services, South West London and St George's Mental Health Services NHS Trust, UK

8.1 Introduction

This chapter covers use of alcohol and illicit drugs in people with intellectual disabilities (see Table 8.1 for definitions). The existing evidence base is discussed and suggestions made for assessment, adapting treatment approaches and working with mainstream services.

There is a paucity of research in substance use in intellectual disabilities, mostly small epidemiological surveys, where inconsistencies in terminology used make for a lack of clarity around level of intellectual disabilities and whether substance use, misuse or disorders are being described.

People with intellectual disabilities may be considered to have less exposure to substances and less opportunity for misuse than the general population but in one study 58.8% of students with intellectual disabilities stated they frequented pubs. These students were found to be knowledgeable about names of alcoholic drinks and their prices and about where and how alcohol could be purchased [1]. Similarly structured interviews of adolescents and university students found those with intellectual disabilities were at least as vulnerable to social influences on alcohol use and abuse but had significantly poorer alcohol-related knowledge than non-disabled peers [2].

The move to community living provides adults with intellectual disabilities greater opportunities to engage in using substances and exposes them to the same stressors of living in modern-day culture that presumably account for the increase in substance use in the general population [3]. The term 'social fragility' has been used to explain substance misuse in the population with intellectual disabilities [4] with both psychological factors and social factors important causally [3]. Psychological factors include reduced self-esteem, loneliness and depression and social factors,

Intellectual Disability Psychiatry: a practical handbook   Angela Hassiotis, Diana Andrea Barron and Ian Hall (eds)
© 2009 John Wiley & Sons, Ltd

Table 8.1 Mental and behavioural disorders due to psychoactive substance use (ICD-10)

- **Acute intoxication.**
- **Harmful use:** A pattern of drinking which has already caused damage to health either physical or mental but does not meet the criteria for dependence.
- **Dependence syndrome:** At least three criteria are present during the past 12 months ranging from withdrawal, impaired control of drinking and use despite harmful consequences to health.
- **Withdrawal.**

Case vignette 8.1

X, a 56-year-old lady with severe intellectual disability, presents with irritability and labile affect every morning at her day centre. She was recently transferred to community living after many years in an institution for people with intellectual disabilities. In the institution she had been prescribed 10 ml of sherry in a medicine cup every night. Staff in her new home misunderstood this and were giving her a large mug of sherry a night.

---

the desire for social acceptance [3]. These predisposing factors for substance misuse mirror those of the wider community.

People with intellectual disabilities and people in the general population who misuse substances seem to be demographically similar in terms of their families and childhood histories, substance use pattern and substance-related problems [5]. There is an overlapping of risk factors between the population with intellectual disabilities as a whole and the general population of people who abuse substances. Risk factors for intellectual disabilities, such as poverty, are also risk factors for substance abuse in the general population. Risk factors for adolescent substance abuse include reduced self-esteem, academic difficulty, loneliness, depression and the desire for social acceptance; all of these are commonly experienced by adolescents with intellectual disabilities. Intellectual disabilities may indirectly lead to substance abuse by generating types of behaviour that lead adolescents to abuse drugs. A poor understanding of one's disability, a lack of skills for developing peer relations and lack of prolonged family support have all been suggested as potential risk factors for substance abuse in intellectual disabilities [6, 7].

Cognitive difficulties experienced by people with intellectual disabilities such as short attention spans, tendencies to distort abstract cognitive concepts and overly compliant dispositions may increase the likelihood of substance use-related problems.

A family history of substance misuse is a risk factor for an individual misusing alcohol and drugs. Furthermore the use of substances, particularly alcohol, during pregnancy can impact on the cognitive development of the fetus. This is exemplified by fetal alcohol syndrome which incorporates cognitive deficits [8, 9]. As a consequence maternal substance misuse can increase the risk of both intellectual disabilities and substance misuse in an individual.

8.2 Range of substances

In groups of people both with and without intellectual disabilities, alcohol is the main substance misused and in both populations levels of substance misuse are increasing. In both populations as substance misuse becomes more common so do the negative consequences to health, social functioning and society. The population of people with intellectual disabilities mirrors the general population in that alcohol and use of illicit drugs tend to co-occur [10].

The prevalence of substance misuse seems to be lower among people with intellectual disabilities than the non-disabled population; one population based study of adults with intellectual disabilities found a prevalence of 1.0% with an incidence of 0.3% [11]. Substance use disorders were commonest in men with mild intellectual disabilities (2.5%) and least common in women with moderate to profound intellectual disabilities (0%). In this study case ascertainment of adults with mild intellectual disabilities was poor so the prevalence of substance use problems in this group may have been underestimated. People with mild intellectual disabilities are often not in contact with intellectual disabilities services and this is a barrier to research into substance use in this population. See Table 8.2

8.3 Alcohol

Structured alcohol questionnaires have in general not been used although the evidence from the general population is that just asking people if they drink is not enough to determine whether they are drinking harmful quantities.

Table 8.2 Substance use in intellectual disabilities

- Less prevalent than in general population
- Older age at first use
- Alcohol use, illicit drug use and smoking co-occur
- More users tend to have substance use disorders than in general population
- More vulnerable to social and psychological consequences of substance use.

Adolescents

Adolescents with intellectual disabilities promised anonymity report higher levels of lifetime alcohol use than those given no such promise, 51% versus 46% in one study [12].

Studies of high school students with intellectual disabilities find lifetime rates of use between 32 and 55% [4, 13] and rates of use in the previous month of 12–39% [7, 12]. All of the studies which compared adolescents with intellectual disabilities with non-disabled peers found higher lifetime and past month prevalence of alcohol use in the non-disabled group [4, 14] but the differences were not large. Those with intellectual disabilities begin drinking later than non-disabled peers [5].

In the general population attention deficit hyperactivity disorder (ADHD) is a major risk factor for development of alcohol use disorders. Most studies report higher rates of ADHD among people with intellectual disabilities than in the general population. ADHD predicts an earlier age of substance dependence onset, a more rapid transition from use to abuse and dependence and longer duration of alcohol use disorder. ADHD with conduct disorder increases the risk of alcohol use disorders; in fact, there is evidence to suggest the relationship between alcohol use disorders and ADHD is primarily mediated by conduct disorder [15]. It seems likely that ADHD in people with intellectual disabilities will increase risks of alcohol use disorders in a similar fashion to the non-disabled population, as the population with intellectual disabilities shares other predictors with the general population. Children with intellectual disabilities and ADHD do not seem to be more likely than children with ADHD alone to develop an alcohol use disorder; in fact, children with higher IQs may be at more risk [16].

> ### Case vignette 8.2
>
> Y is a 22-year-old man with mild intellectual disability who presents via the criminal justice system after inappropriate behaviour towards a female at a bus station while intoxicated with alcohol and cannabis. At interview, psychosis is diagnosed. In his past history he had ADHD diagnosed in childhood. He stopped prescribed medication at 18 and began using substances. He now presents with harmful use of drugs and alcohol. An offence history of stealing to obtain substances predates the presenting offence.

Adults

The prevalence of alcohol use amongst those with intellectual disabilities lies between 39 and 52%, with 33% reporting weekly drinking [13]. The prevalence of alcohol use disorders lies between 0.5 and 2% of the intellectual disabilities population with

7% of these drinking every day [13]. Adults with intellectual disabilities who use alcohol also often use illicit drugs, with one study finding one-fifth of alcohol users also using combinations of illicit drugs (cannabis, ecstasy, amphetamines) and/or prescribed medication [10].

There is some evidence that although the prevalence of alcohol use disorders is lower, the rate of problem drinking among drinkers is greater in those with a intellectual disability [17]. suggesting that people with intellectual disabilities may have a lower threshold for alcohol-related problems requiring less alcohol [5]. This is similar in those with severe mental health problems who may not fulfil the criteria for dependence but still experience significant levels of psychological and social harm at lower levels of substance use than the general population.

There is also evidence that alcohol misusing adults with intellectual disabilities experience alcohol-related social consequences at a level that is equivalent to if not higher than that experienced in the general population: increased levels of psychological, family and social problems have been reported with high rates of job-related and legal consequences [13].

Alcohol use disorders in adults with intellectual disabilities seem to have a chronic course with one study finding for over 75% alcohol misuse had continued for over five years despite attempts at treatment [10].

8.4 Drugs

Adolescents

Adolescents with intellectual disabilities promised anonymity report higher rates of illicit drug use than those given no such promise: marijuana 29% versus 5%, cocaine 3% versus 0% and other illicit drugs 7% versus 0% [12]. Adolescents with intellectual disabilities report much lower rates of illicit drug use than non-disabled peers in every study bar one, which found 70% of students with a chemical dependency had an intellectual disability [18]. Reports of lifetime use of marijuana vary from 13 to 26%, while past month use of marijuana varies from 4 to 10% [12, 13]. Lifetime use of other drugs seems to be low (cocaine 3%) and monthly rates of other drug use extremely low [4, 12].

Adults

There seems to be a much lower prevalence than in the general population and illicit drug use seems to be commonly associated with alcohol misuse. Of those who do use illicit drugs a significant percentage (one third in one study) show harmful use or dependence and the consequences in terms of family, psychological and social problems are at least as severe, if not more severe, than those experienced by non-disabled populations [5, 13].

8.5 Assessment

Within the general population alcohol and drug use disorders are missed in certain groups such as:

- younger patients

- high risk groups such as hospital inpatients and people with mental health problems

- people drinking at harmful levels (1 in 80 identified) and

- people with alcohol dependency (1 in 28 identified).

Substance use disorders are missed in the population with intellectual disabilities too: we may be embarrassed to ask about substance use or may discount its possibility.

Health professionals working with people with intellectual disabilities need to be careful not to misattribute symptoms of substance abuse, such as irritability, to the intellectual disability itself (see Table 8.3: identifying substance abuse).

Cognitive and communication difficulties may challenge our history taking.

Problems with temporal recall may make answering questions about how much was drunk in the past week, month or year difficult. Numeracy problems are common so questions about number of drinks and the concept of units of alcohol are problematic. More abstract questions, such as questions about not doing things normally expected of you because of your substance use, are often not understood. Questions may assume a pre-existing knowledge base that people with intellectual disabilities do not possess, for example questions about blackouts in alcohol use.

People with intellectual disabilities may not know that too much alcohol can be harmful or even that alcohol causes intoxication. They may not be aware of that there is alcohol in certain drinks such as 'Alco pops'. They may not make the expected cognitive links, for example they may blame being intoxicated on the alcohol and not on themselves for drinking it. Similarly substance abusers are commonly asked if they want help but people with intellectual disabilities may be unaware of the problems

Table 8.3   Identifying substance abuse

- Ask all service users and carers about substance abuse.
- Be aware of high risk groups (young men with mild or borderline IQs, ADHD and conduct disorder, adolescents with ADHD who smoke and those with mental health problems).
- Look for substance abuse associated behavioural or physical problems; consider urine and blood tests.

---

that their abuse may cause and may need education about this before being able to say whether or not they want help; indeed they may have no concept of abuse. Assessors may rely on collateral histories but people with intellectual disabilities may conceal substance use from carers or parents and informants may not have full information.

It is also important to remember that alcohol and drugs give pleasurable effects and making the link between both euphoria and the adverse impact of a substance for a person with intellectual impairment may be more difficult than for the general population. Screening questionnaires such as the CAGE and AUDIT for alcohol, though not validated in the intellectual disabled population, may be helpful in identifying alcohol-related disorders, though consideration may need to be made of the language used. See Table 8.4 for advice on taking an alcohol history in intellectual disability.

The challenges of history taking make an awareness of risk factors, the consequences of substance use in intellectual disabilities, comorbidity and vulnerability factors important:

1. **Risk factors for alcohol use disorders are:** being male, young; having a borderline or mild intellectual disability; living independently; having a mental health problem; problem behaviours, [10, 11, 19] smoking, especially in adolescents with ADHD, and ADHD especially if associated with conduct disorder.
2. **The main consequences of substance misuse in adults with intellectual disabilities are:** verbal and physical aggression; erratic mood changes; suicidal ideation; rows with carers; vulnerability to exploitation; offending behaviour, injuring self and attending A&E [10].
3. **Comorbidity with mental health:** in the general population 8–15% of patients of community mental health teams and 49% of psychiatric inpatients have alcohol use disorders. People with intellectual disabilities have an increased prevalence of mental illness. One study [11] found no association between substance use disorder and mental illness, but another found 33% of 41 participants had a co-existing mental health problem [10]. See Table 8.5: alcohol use disorders and psychiatric disorder can co-occur.
4. **Criminality:** ADHD with conduct disorder increases the risk of alcohol use disorders. There is a strong link between ADHD, alcohol use disorders and criminality. This link is particularly strong in individuals with both ADHD and conduct disorder [15]. Alcohol or drug misuse has been associated with admission to secure hospital facilities in non-psychotic people with intellectual disabilities [20].
5. **Gambling:** may be associated [10].
6. **Vulnerability/predisposing factors (look for in history):** Within the general population adults with histories of sexual abuse have increased rates of alcohol problems and people with intellectual disabilities are vulnerable to such abuse. See Table 8.6. A family history of substance abuse seems to predispose people with intellectual disabilities to abuse substances [5].

Table 8.4 Taking an alcohol history from a person with intellectual disability

- Aim to see without carer and reassure the interview is confidential.
- Ask what they drink then ask how many they had at any one time (i.e. the most).
- Then ask if this is usually what they drink and if not ask how it is different.
- Ask to see the bottle or can or show pictures of drinks.
- Ask about drinking in the previous week; go through it day by day asking what they did each day as well as whether they drank.
- Then ask was this a usual week or not; if not ask about a usual week.
- Establish past events (recent first then more distant) that are significant to them and that they remember and then ask them to recall whether they were drinking then to try and establish changes in drinking over time and periods of abstinence.
- Ask their view on why they drink.
- Ask: Do they think drinking is good or bad? and ask them to explain their answer.
- Ask whether family and people around them drink. Do their friends drink? Have people around them said anything about their drinking?
- Ask: Are they the same or different when they drink? If they say different, ask them to explain.
- Ask: Have you been recently angry, had arguments or got into trouble or hurt yourself? If they say yes, ask if they had a drink or no drink when this happened. Ask: Do they think the drink made them angry? and so on.
- Ask: Do you think drink has changed your memory? Better or worse?
- In asking about withdrawal symptoms, physical symptoms, may be better recounted than psychological ones so ask about physical symptoms (tremor, sweating, nausea, anxiety, particularly on waking) in detail.
- In asking about craving give examples; try and pick situations from the context of the history they have given you so if they always drink in the local pub ask them about walking past the pub, if they drink at home ask about seeing drink on TV. Try and avoid the word 'if'. Ask: Do you want a drink? Then ask: Is it a small want or a big want? Then ask: Can you ignore the feeling or not?
- Ask what they have spent their money on in the last week. Then ask: Is this is usual or different?
- Ask them what they know about alcohol (effects, safe limits). Then ask: Do you think your drinking is OK or too much?
- Ask: If you stop drinking, will your life be the same or different? If different, ask them to explain.
- Do ask: Do you want help with drinking? But remember they may need basic education about alcohol before they know enough to know they need help.
- Collateral histories are important.

Table 8.5 Alcohol use disorders and psychiatric disorder can co-occur as

---

- Primary mental illness with subsequent alcohol use disorders
- Primary alcohol use disorders with psychiatric sequelae
- Dual primary diagnosis.

Table 8.6 Brief intervention for people with intellectual disabilities

---

- Keep it simple
- Ask the user how much they drink. The recommended limits are 14 units per week for woman and 21 units per week for men; 1 unit is usually equivalent to about 0.5 standard glass of wine, 0.5 pint beer or 1 measure of spirits [21].
- Advise no more than three drinks at a time and at least two abstinent days per week.
- Support verbal advice with appropriate information, for example BILD booklet on alcohol and smoking 1998.

> **Case vignette 8.3**
>
> T is a 24-year-old woman with mild intellectual disability who had a deprived and abusive upbringing with sexual abuse both from her stepfather and at her residential school. She presents via the criminal justice system having stolen whiskey from a supermarket at the instruction of her boyfriend. Her boyfriend has been supplying her with crack cocaine in exchange for her prostituting herself for him. She is on the point of eviction from her residential care home because of stealing and illicit drug use. She has limited numeracy and literacy. She is found not to be fit to plead and transferred to a medium secure unit for women with intellectual disabilities for assessment.

8.6 Adapting treatment approaches

People with intellectual disabilities may have very limited knowledge; they may not know alcohol causes intoxication or harm and find concepts like safe limits or units of alcohol difficult to understand. Alcohol education programmes start at too high a level and available materials may not be appropriate. The result is that it may be more difficult for people with intellectual disabilities to move through the stages of change which rely on an increasing awareness of one's problem and developing an internal locus of control. People with intellectual disabilities may struggle to develop an internal locus of control because their life experience has been one of limited control and responsibility. They may struggle to link actions and consequences, for example that drinking again will result in a return to old behaviours and problems.

The issue of capacity may be raised when an adult with intellectual disability's addictive behaviour is putting them, or others, at risk and they do not seem to have a sufficient understanding or ability to retain or weigh up or use information around risks in making decisions about their substance use. Care needs to be taken to distinguish bad decision making from lack of capacity. Care also needs to be taken to distinguish lack of capacity from an impairment or disturbance in functioning of the person's mind owing to their intellectual disabilities and cognitive distortions resulting from addiction. The former, if sufficient to render the person unable to make decisions, suggests grounds to proceed as per the Mental Capacity Act and the latter does not. In practice it may be difficult to make the distinction. This is an area that can be fraught with heightened emotions and although in law people with intellectual disabilities are allowed to make bad decisions in practice those around them tend to be reluctant to allow this to happen when substance abuse is involved and will take steps, for example to remove financial control from them or to move them to more supported accommodation.

In the general population brief advice and intervention result in one in eight patients who are drinking at harmful levels moderating their drinking to low-risk levels. People with intellectual disabilities can moderate their drinking in response to verbal advice combined with appropriate information, for example the BILD booklet on alcohol and smoking, 1998 (see Table 8.7).

Adults with intellectual disabilities may have reduced literacy, be slower learners and have short-term memory deficits so treatment strategies need to be adapted to meet their needs. Various adaptations have been suggested including lengthening the treatment period, frequent repetition, use of role play and discussions and demonstrations of inappropriate behaviours [13].

Table 8.7 Epilepsy and alcohol abuse

- Check blood levels of antiepileptic drugs which are metabolized through the liver.
- Remember alcohol use as a reason for increases in seizure frequency.
- If drinking at high levels, advise not to stop suddenly as this can precipitate seizures in both epileptic and non-epileptic people.
- Benzodiazepines can affect plasma concentration of phenytoin.
- Valproate increases plasma concentration of diazepam and lorazepam.
- Disulfiram inhibits metabolism of phenytoin.

Assertiveness training and modelling interventions have both been found to be effective in increasing substance knowledge and enhancing skills in adults with intellectual disabilities but neither intervention was superior to delayed treatment on measures of substance abuse [13].

Motivational interviewing is a powerful cognitive behavioural technique to deal with ambivalence in people with alcohol use disorders. It has been successfully adapted to adults with intellectual disabilities with increases in patients' motivation, self-efficacy and determination to change drinking behaviour [22].

Comorbidity, cognitive and communication difficulties and increased prevalence of epilepsy suggest operating a lower threshold for admitting people with intellectual disabilities who are withdrawing from alcohol. See Tables 8.8 and 8.9 on epilepsy and alcohol abuse; managing ADHD and alcohol use disorders.

Case vignette 8.4

L is a 22-year-old man with a mild intellectual disability working as a cleaner. He presented to addiction services, drinking 20 pints of wine or beer daily and experiencing alcohol withdrawal symptoms as well as auditory hallucinations related to this. In addition he was diagnosed with epilepsy two years prior to his presentation. Initially he was considered for inpatient detoxification from alcohol, but managed to cut down and achieve abstinence prior to this. L engaged well with AA and found the mentoring process and 12 steps very helpful. He also attended counselling for his alcohol use provided by local voluntary agencies. L has had occasional relapse bingeing on alcohol but he is no longer drinking daily in a dependent manner.

Table 8.8 Managing ADHD and alcohol use disorders

- Psychostimulants can be safe and effective.
- Untreated ADHD may hinder treatment of alcohol use disorders.
- Try non-stimulant medications first.
- Multidisciplinary team assessment and risk benefit analysis prior to using stimulant.
- Use sustained release preparations and monitor carefully.
- Discontinue if alcohol use disorder worsens or evidence of diversion of prescribed medication.

Table 8.9 Adults with alcohol use disorders who have been sexually abused compared to those who have not been abused are:

- Younger
- Have family histories of alcohol misuse
- Have more alcohol-related problems.

8.7 Working with mainstream and voluntary services

When people with mild intellectual disabilities develop substance use problems they may come into contact with mainstream addictions services where they have described their contacts in negative terms and where their mild intellectual disabilities may be missed [10]. In general people with intellectual disabilities may find accessing substance misuse services difficult and tend to present to intellectual disability services. They may find sessions difficult to follow or that information assumes too high a level of pre-existing knowledge. Substance misuse workers may not have any training or experience in working with people with intellectual disabilities, and mainstream intellectual disabilities services may similarly struggle to manage issues around substance use [23]. People with intellectual disabilities may be blamed for failing when in fact the substance missue programme has failed them. People with intellectual disabilities may be excluded from group programmes or find integrating into (Narcotics Anonymous (NA) or Alcoholics Anonymous (AA) difficult. However most 12-step programmes encourage wide access so people particularly those with mild intellectual disabilities may benefit from both AA and NA. The ethos of mainstream substance use services, that users are responsible and help is given when users are contemplating change, maybe at odds with the lack of control and responsibility people with intellectual disabilities are given in their lives.

Joint working to combine the expertise of community addictions and intellectual disability teams is probably the best way to meet the needs of a person with intellectual disabilities who has a substance use disorder. Community addictions teams will assess and allocate a key worker. They know about local voluntary organizations and how to access them. Some areas have specialist workers who work across community intellectual disability teams and community addictions teams. One example is the specialist social worker for drug and alcohol problems in southwest London who provides liaison between local community intellectual disabilities and addictions services and additional resources tailored to the needs of adults with intellectual disabilities, such as one-to-one work.

References

1. Buttimer, J. and Tierney, E. (2005) Patterns of leisure participation among adolescents with a mild intellectual disability. *Journal of Intellectual Disabilities*, **9** (1), 25–42.

2. McCusker, C.G., Clare, I.C.H., Cullen, C. and Reep, J. (1993) Alcohol-related knowledge and attitudes in people with a mild learning disability. *Journal of Community and Applied Social Psychology*, **3**, 29–40.

3. Taggart, L., McLaughlin, D. and Quinn, B. (2007) Listening to people with learning disabilities who misuse alcohol and drugs. *Health and Social Care in the Community*, **15** (4), 360–368.

4. Gress, J.R. and Boss, M.R. (1996) Substance abuse differences among students receiving special education school services. *Child Psychiatry Human Development*, **26**, 235–246.

5. Westermeyer, J., Kemp, K. and Nugent, S. (1988) Substance use and abuse among mentally retarded persons: a comparison of patients and a survey population. *American Journal of Drug and Alcohol Abuse*, **14**, 109–123.

6. Cosden, M. (2001) Risk and resilience for substance abuse among adolescents and adults with learning disabilities. *Journal of Learning Disabilities*, **34** (4), 352–358.

7. Emerson, E. and Turnbull, L. (2005) Self-reported smoking and alcohol use among adolescents with intellectual disabilities. *Journal of Intellectual Disabilities*, **9**, 58–69.

8. Lemoine, P., Harouseau, H., Borteryu, J.T. and Menuet, J.C. (1968) Les enfants des parents alcooliques; anomalies observees apropos de 127 cas. *Oeust Medical*, **21**, 476–482.

9. Jones, K.L. and Smith, D.W. (1973) Recognition of the fetal alcohol syndrome in early pregnancy. *Lancet*, **2**, 999–1001.

10. Taggart, L., McLaughlin, D., Quinn, B. and Milligan, V. (2006) An exploration of substance misuse in people with intellectual disabilities. *Journal of Intellectual Disabilities and Research*, **50** (8), 588–597.

11. Cooper, S.A., Smiley, E., Morrison, J. *et al.* (2007) Mental ill-health in adults with intellectual disabilities: prevalence and associated factors. *British Journal of Psychiatry*, **190**, 27–35.

12. Pack, R., Wallander, J.L. and Browne, D. (1998) Health risk behaviours of African American adolescents with mild mental retardation: prevalence depends on measurement method. *American Journal of Mental Retardation*, **102**, 409–420.

13. McGillicuddy, N. (2006) A review of substance use research among those with mental retardation. *Mental Retardation and Developmental Disabilities Research Reviews*, **12**, 41–47.

14. Blum, R.W., Kelly, A. and Ireland, M. (2001) Health risk behaviours and protective factors among adolescents with mobility impairments and learning and emotional disabilities. *Journal of Adolescent Health*, **28**, 481–490.

15. Levin, R. (2007) ADHD and substance abuse update. *American Journal of Addictions*, **16**, 1–4.

16. Molina, B.S.G. and Pellham, W.E. (2001) Substance use, substance abuse, and LD among adolescents with a childhood history of ADHD. *Journal of Learning Disabilities*, **34**, 333–334.

17. Degenhardt, L. (2000) Interventions for people with alcohol use disorders and an intellectual disability: a review of the literature. *Journal of Intellectual and Developmental Disability*, **25**, 135–146.
18. Karacostas, D.D. and Fisher, G.L. (1993) Chemical dependency in students with and without learning disabilities. *Journal of Learning Disabilities*, **26**, 491–495.
19. Barrett, N. and Paschos, D. (2006) Alcohol-related problems in adolescents with intellectual disabilities. *Current Opinion in Psychiatry*, **19** (5), 481–485.
20. Doody, G.A., Thomson, L.D.G., Miller, P. and Johnstone, E,C. (2001) Predictors of admission to a high-security hospital of people with intellectual disability with and without schizophrenia. *Journal of Intellectual Disability Research*, **44** (2), 130.
21. Department of Health (2008) http://www.dh.gov.uk/en/Publichealth/Healthimprovement/Alcoholmisuse/DH_085385.
22. Mendel, E. and Hipkins, J. (2002) Motivating learning disabled offenders with alcohol-related problems: a pilot study. *British Journal of Learning Disabilities*, **30** (4), 153–158.
23. McLaughlin, D.F., Taggart, L., Quinn, B. and Milligan, V. (2007) The experiences of professionals who care for people with intellectual disability who have substance related problems. *Journal of Substance Use*, **12** (2), 133–143.

Further reading

BILD Booklet on Alcohol and Smoking, (1998), www.bild.org.uk/03books_health.htm10Your GoodHealth.

Miller, H. (2008) Alcohol use disorders, in *The Frith Prescribing Guidelines For Adults with Intellectual Disability*, Chapter 18 (eds S. Bhaumik and D. Brandford), HealthComm UK Ltd, pp. 191–198.

Kranzler, H. and Ciraulo, D. (eds) (2005) *Clinical Manual of Addiction Psychopharmacology*, American Psychiatric Publishing Inc.

9 Challenging Behaviour

David Smith[1] and William Howie[2]

[1]CAMHS, South West London and St George's Mental Health NHS Trust, London, UK
[2]Assessment and Intervention Team, South West London and St George's Mental Health NHS Trust, London, UK

9.1 Introduction

Definitions of challenging behaviour

Challenging behaviour is a social construct and has been defined by Emerson as:

> *culturally abnormal behaviour(s) of such intensity, frequency or duration that the physical safety of the person or others is likely to be put in jeopardy, or behaviour which is likely to limit the use of, or result in the person being denied access to ordinary community facilities [1].*

To include a developmental perspective the Mental Health Foundation have added 'or impair a child's growth, development or family life . . . ' [2]

Concept of challenging behaviour

Clements and Zarkowska state there is 'no generally accepted list of behaviours to which we automatically attach this label. It is a social judgement, not an objective scientific diagnosis' [3]. This distinction is frequently misunderstood and overlooked; a behaviour that is challenging to one person or service may, to another, be understood as a form of self-expression.

The term challenging behaviour 'challenges' the people controlling the individual's environment to make a systematic attempt to understand the meaning of the behaviour in context and to meet the individual's needs. It is potentially more worrying that a person might fail to communicate serious needs.

Intellectual Disability Psychiatry: a practical handbook   Angela Hassiotis, Diana Andrea Barron and Ian Hall (eds)
© 2009 John Wiley & Sons, Ltd

A limitation of this concept is that it can be effectively applied only to those who are classed by society as not being responsible for their behaviour. This is important when considering the relationship between challenging and offending behaviour. Describing behaviour as challenging rather than criminal implies evidence that the person lacks understanding that would otherwise render them accountable. Offending behaviour is covered in Chapter 12.

Prevalence of challenging behaviour in people with learning disabilities

Emerson and colleagues have reviewed prevalence [4] noting that the prevalence of challenging behaviour within the intellectual disability population is difficult to calculate and depends on methodology used for defining challenging behaviour. Previous studies focus on either aggression or self-injury, often using unrepresentative populations. The subjective nature of the concept complicates quantifying, with recent estimates varying in finding that between 1.91 and 6.33 people per 10 000 of the general population have challenging behaviour in the context of an intellectual disability [1, 4–6].

Aetiology of challenging behaviour

Generally challenging behaviour represents a communication of the individual's needs, whether intentionally or unintentionally. We stress the importance of communication as central for understanding and managing challenging behaviour (communication is further addressed in Chapter 2). That behaviour has been labelled as challenging may reflect lack of resources and the label may reflect the needs of the network rather than the individual.

Aggressive and self-injurious behaviours have often been considered an innate part of a person's presentation, without consideration of alternative explanations, an idea called *diagnostic overshadowing*.

The presentation may have physical, psychological or social underpinnings or a combination of the three and these may impact on treatment and management strategies. The specific and wide ranging aetiologies underpinning challenging behaviour are discussed further in the sections dealing with assessment below.

9.2 Systemic perspectives in challenging behaviour

The thinking that underlies the concept of challenging behaviour and even the choice of the term is fundamentally systemic [7]. The idea that the problem resides within a system and not just within an individual opens up new ways of thinking and working. The person exists in context, and understanding context facilitates understanding the person and their actions.

Case vignette 9.1

George is a 40-year-old man with diabetes who attends a day centre. George has recently been reported to be throwing objects during the ceramics class. Perhaps poor diabetic control is contributing to observed behaviour, but that does not explain why the behaviour is happening at that time. Maybe George is copying other people, but because George has a reputation, carers notice his behaviour and label it as inappropriate. However, that does not explain why the behaviour has been brought to attention at this particular time. George might be reflecting changes outside the day centre. Without understanding George's life in context, important factors may be overlooked.

Language is important and can promote and perpetuate disadvantage experienced by people with disabilities and their families. Everyday words like 'normal' can cause confusion and distress by implying that the individual with an intellectual disability is abnormal. A terminology that acknowledges the humanity of the individual is encouraged. We avoid terms that label the individual as the problem even at the expense of brevity. Careful practitioners try to acknowledge problems without blaming or marginalizing the individual and their family or network of support.

The systemic perspective explicitly acknowledges the social context of disability and stigma. Carers may have an acute awareness of the socio-political context of disability and processes of marginalization.

Systemic thinking is commonly called family therapy. However the term family therapy neglects the system outside the family. 'Therapy' implies issues needing treatment, which might attribute blame to the family and add to their burden, whereas 'systemic thinking' acknowledges the wider socio-political context. Modern systemic thinking acknowledges strengths in individuals and network, and highlights and enhances abilities, de-emphasizing therapist expertise. Professionals can help families recognize their own skills and strengths. Thinking of parents and carers as *co-therapists* aids collaboration.

Systemic thinking incorporates valuable techniques and provides a framework for understanding. The idea that the solution is more useful than the problem underlies moves to improve quality of life for all, with initiatives like person centred planning and health action plans. If a behaviour is absent in certain situations, then those situations may tell us more about the answers than any amount of analysis.

Valuing of diversity is another important idea, whether related to ability, gender, culture, race, age or sexuality.

Socio-political context

Mansell emphasizes the role of commissioning specialist services in managing challenging behaviour [8, in 17]. Clinicians have a role in advocating for adequate resources as well as focussing on individual situations.

9.3 Assessment

Introduction

Much time is spent trying to understand the motivations behind challenging behaviour, and this can be a technical and demanding process. However, understanding the physical and mental health needs along with the social context is also important. The assessment should be proportionate to the problem aiming to quickly identify remediable situations, treatable conditions and excluding serious medical conditions.

Case vignette 9.2

Barbara has been banging her head against the floor. Urine testing reveals an infection. She receives antibiotics and pain relief and 24 hours later the head-banging stops. The putative underlying cause was readily established and successfully treated.

Cursory investigation may not provide a clear understanding of the situation. For more complex cases deeper understanding of the individual in the context of their life and their system underpins successful management. A thorough process of assessment will usually require multiple interviews of the index patient, their family and carers and professionals in their network. Physical assessment with investigations often reveals useful information.

Diagnosis: physical and mental health assessment

Challenging behaviour is not a diagnosis, but a diagnosis may inform management. Challenging behaviour often reflects an underlying physical problem that the person has been unable to communicate or it may be a manifestation of an underlying mental disorder. Physical and mental disorders are often more common in people with intellectual disabilities and the morbidity and mortality in this patient group remain higher than in the general population [4] (Table 9.1).

Table 9.1 Common physical and mental disorders associated with challenging behaviour

Diagnosed physical complaints	Dental pain
	Urinary tract infections
	Respiratory infections
	Gastritis/gastric ulceration
	Constipation
Presumptive physical complaints	Pyrexia without evidence of localized infection
	Gastro-oesophageal reflux
	Gastritis
	Headache
Diagnosed mental disorders	Anxiety disorders
	Depressive disorders
	Psychotic disorders
	Insomnia
	Hyperkinetic disorder
	Autistic disorders
Presumptive mental disorders and sub-syndromal conditions	Anxiety
	Apparent distress
	Inattentiveness

A physical condition presenting as challenging behaviour may be life threatening and may be readily treated, so investigating remediable causes is a priority. There may still be an acute problem even in chronic challenging behaviour.

Simple observation and measurement of body functioning, such as weight, temperature, pulse, blood pressure and respiratory rate, can suggest a cause and rule out many of the more worrying conditions. An assessment of sight and hearing may be informative, particularly if conditions associated with sensory impairment such as Down's syndrome are present.

Mental disorders, particularly depressive disorders, are more common in people with intellectual disabilities, but limitations in communication and reliance on third-party information can result in standard diagnostic criteria, such as, ICD-10 not being reached. The development of specific criteria for people with intellectual disabilities – the Diagnostic Criteria for People with Learning Disabilities [9] (DC-LD) reflects this challenge.

Neurodevelopmental disorders

Neurodevelopmental disorders is being used here to refer to a range of conditions where there is an uneven profile of performance over the range of higher intellectual functioning. In addition to autistic disorders and attention deficit disorders (ADDs) included in some narrow definitions, all conditions believed to have a biological basis including behavioural phenotypes are included. Assessment of individual behaviours benefits from knowledge of characteristic patterns of behaviour associated with neurodevelopmental disorders.

Challenging behaviour is more likely to arise in situations where the individual's needs are not understood by the systems supporting them. A person centred approach (see Chapter 2) is central to working with people with intellectual disabilities; however, often assumptions undermine this. One common assumption is that the expressive verbal ability indicates overall performance. Both overestimation and underestimation can cause problems.

Case vignette 9.3

Some people with cerebral palsy have dysarthria and may become frustrated when people underestimate their receptive ability. Conversely some people with foetal alcohol syndrome may have relatively good verbal fluency but less good sequencing skills, leaving carers confused when they struggle when others of similar verbal fluency do not.

Behavioural phenotypes

The recognized patterns of behaviour associated with conditions of known aetiology, called behavioural phenotypes, help to predict and understand a person's particular strengths and difficulties.

Definition of behavioural phenotype:

A characteristic pattern of motor, cognitive, linguistic and/or social abnormalities which is consistently associated with a biological disorder.

OR ... a heightened probability that people with a given syndrome will exhibit behavioral or developmental sequelae relative to others without the syndrome.

A number of conditions are associated with high levels of worrying behaviours including self-injurious and aggressive behaviour and the behaviour can be quite stereotyped (Table 9.2).

Table 9.2 Conditions with associated specific behaviours

Lesch–Nyhan syndrome	Lip biting
Smith Magenis syndrome	Pulling out finger and toe nails
Prader Willi syndrome	Hyperphagia

Autistic spectrum disorders

Autistic spectrum disorders (ASDs) are a group of disorders where understanding the impact of the condition on the individual is likely to improve management (see also Chapter 7). Autism is an important focus in challenging behaviour. The triad of impaired communication, difficulties in social interaction and restricted, repetitive behaviour characterize autism. Historically autism was narrowly defined, but more recently the idea of a spectrum of disorder (ASD) or a group of related disorders (e.g. pervasive developmental disorders) has improved the recognition of the needs of a much larger population who have similar needs. All of the main symptom areas can be a useful focus of clinical attention, and recognizing a pervasive developmental disorder can guide clinicians to look for other problems. These include hypersensitivity, particularly to sound, problems with eating and sleeping, and common comorbid mental disorders such as depression. The restricted interests, problems with communication and difficulty with managing social situations may all complicate learning.

Although valuable generalizations can be made about people with ASD, heterogeneity must also be acknowledged, challenging assumptions that because a diagnosis has been made the person will behave in a particular fashion.

Attention deficit disorders

Attention deficit disorders (ADDs) are a group of conditions that have had much public attention in recent years particularly around controversies about the use of medication such as methylphenidate. Although both inattention and hyperactivity are important components in the conditions, hyperactivity tends to be more evident and indeed in ICD-10 the condition is known as hyperkinetic disorder.

Although associated with childhood, they may persist into adulthood. The inattentive presentation may be missed in females, older children and adults. Stimulant medication and second line medications may improve concentration and subsequently behaviour. Unfortunately there is considerable comorbidity and medication alone is unlikely to meet the needs of the person fully.

Verbal/performance mismatch

Within a range of conditions significant differences in verbal and performance abilities complicate understanding. Some people find difficulty completing tasks that their verbal fluency would suggest they were capable of undertaking. Cognitive testing may reveal that verbal ability outperforms other areas of cognitive functioning. This information can be used to help the person's support network to understand that the individual is not misbehaving but trying to conform within the limits of their ability. Challenging behaviour in this case reflects a problem in the carer's excessive expectations, reflecting the value of a concept that does not centre pathology in the individual.

Multiple diagnoses

The presence of an aetiological diagnosis such as a genetic condition does not preclude a phenomenological diagnosis such as an ASD and indeed a number of conditions are associated with other neurodevelopmental disorders (Table 9.3). Diagnosis and factual information about the incidence of these behaviours in these conditions can help families and carers not to feel responsible for the person's apparent distress.

9.4 Functional assessment

Immediate action to minimize risks is often required, particularly with self-injury or aggression. Having contained immediate risks, further attempts to stop, minimize or change the behaviour are based on a detailed assessment aiming to understand the purpose the behaviour serves. This information can be used to replace it, where possible, with a behaviour serving the same purpose. The functional assessment process examines the individual, their environment and their functioning to understand the behaviour and what it means for the client.

Table 9.3 Examples of conditions associated with neurodevelopmental disorders

Fragile X syndrome	ASD, ADD
Tuberous sclerosis	ASD

Ball, Bush and Emerson [10] propose a six-step approach to assessment when working with people who exhibit challenging behaviour including:

1. pre-assessment
2. assessment
3. formulation
4. intervention
5. evaluation
6. feedback.

Functional assessment is an iterative process that develops as the assessment progresses and continues as treatments are offered, implemented and their effectiveness measured. In the document *Challenging Behaviour: A Unified Approach* [10] a three-stage approach is presented that includes hypothesis development, testing and refining.

Gathering information

Gathering information is the first part of a functional assessment. As well as collecting biographical data it is also important to collect information about the client and associated problems. This might include reports from other professionals working with the client such as psychologists, psychiatrists, speech and language therapists and the general practitioner. Information from these sources may reveal the history of the problem behaviour and what interventions, behavioural or otherwise, have been tried with the client in the past. This data allows the professional to establish who is involved with the client and who and what needs to be involved in the assessment and the format the assessment might take.

Interview

A detailed interview with those closest to the client and sometimes with the client is often invaluable. This may include parents and other carers, college or day centre staff and paid carers. Interviews with these people will help the professional clarify the behaviours and gain information about what is of most concern and its impact on the client and others. A number of formats for conducting detailed interviews are available including a comprehensive one by O'Neill *et al.* [11]. that looks at behaviour in detail and ends with the possible formulation or hypothesis (summary statements) about the function of the behaviour that can then lead to the next stage of the assessment process. The O'Neill interview includes a detailed look at the possible antecedents to the target behaviour, including communication, diet, sleep and physical health. Interviews effectively obtain detailed information about a client and the problems but rely on the skill of the interviewer and the openness of the interviewee.

Direct observation and baseline data

Baseline data show what is happening prior to treatment taking place. It might include the frequency of the behaviour, the duration of each episode of behaviour and the times of the day the behaviour happens as well as information about the antecedents and consequences of behaviour. This data is invaluable at later stages in the assessment and in the treatment phase and will allow the clinician to measure the effectiveness of interventions by measuring frequency or duration of behaviour post-treatment against that collected during baseline phase.

Antecedents, behaviour and consequences (ABC)

Looking at the antecedents (what is happening before the behaviour occurs) and consequences (what happens after the behaviour) of behaviour is essential in determining what the function of the behaviour might be. This method of data collection can be completed by the professional undertaking the assessment, and with some instruction, by parents and others carers who know the client. This portion of the functional assessment allows a better understanding of the environment the client inhabits, including the physical environment, and routines as well as what might be triggering or reinforcing the behaviour.

Zarkowska and Clements [12] use a four-stage process that focuses on the settings, triggers, action and response (STAR). They look closely at the environment where the behaviour takes place and encourage looking at wider environmental factors including the temperature, the number of people, any demands being made on the client, noise levels, routines, choices and opportunities and so on.

Both models require a description of the behaviour that is observable and measurable.

Frequency and duration

Data regarding the frequency and duration of the behaviour are an essential part of the baseline measurement. As with the antecedents, behaviour and consequences (ABCs) or STAR analysis it is important to have a description of the behaviour that is observable and measurable so that everyone is recording the same (target) behaviour. Frequency recording is simple to do and requires the observer to count the number of times a behaviour happens over a given period of time; this can be done either using mechanical devices such as tally counters or simply placing a tick on a page.

Some behaviours are difficult to count as discrete events because they not only happen but often last for long periods of time, for example sleeping. A record of duration is the most meaningful way to measure these. To complete duration recording the total length of time the client engages in the behaviour is recorded. The easiest way to do this is with a stopwatch where either the time of each episode is recorded or the total amount of time spent engaging in the behaviour is recorded. For behaviour that happens infrequently it may be necessary to complete interval or time-sampling recordings where the presence or absence of the target behaviour in a particular period of time is noted.

Frequency and duration recordings are simple and cheap to complete and, provided there is a good working definition of the target behaviour, can be completed by clinicians and by parents and carers. Good frequency data is important in looking at the spread of the behaviour over the client's day or over a longer period of time.

The collection of data; ABC, frequency and duration, should be collected over a period of time and in a number of different environments so that a true representation of the behaviour, or absence of behaviour, is obtained.

Questionnaires

A number of questionnaires are available for the clinician to use as part of the functional assessment including the Motivation Assessment Scale [13] and the Questions About Behavioral Function [14]. Both of these questionnaires look at the possible communicatory function of challenging behaviour (attention maintained, demand avoidance, access to tangible items, etc.). Both use Likert scales and between 16 and 26 questions to determine the major function(s) of the behaviour. Both questionnaires are quick and easy to complete and can be completed by anyone who knows the client and has seen the client display the target behaviour. For a detailed look at assessment schedules see O'Brien et al. [15].

Data analysis and formulation

After completion of the pre-assessment work, detailed interview and direct obser-vation of the client, the information and data collected needs to be analysed and formulated.

At the end of the formulation it should be possible to put forward a hypothesis, or summary statement, of why the behaviour happens, when it happens, in what situations it occurs and the variables that control it. This might then lead on to an intervention (such as those discussed under 'management' below) or to further assessment and analysis. If it is not clear at this stage what the function of the behaviour is, it may be necessary to complete further assessment including manipulations (detailed assessment that controls the antecedents and consequences of the behaviour and is sometimes known as analog assessment).

9.5 Management

The vast majority of challenging behaviour is managed successfully in the community. This is our main focus in the discussion of management. Effective management of challenging behaviour usually requires understanding the behaviour in the context in which it arises. Admission to hospital or specialist challenging behaviour unit can prevent the development of this understanding by taking the individual out of their familiar context.

Community treatment of challenging behaviour

There are more than 12 000 people with an intellectual disability and challenging behaviour living in the community in the UK [16] in a variety of settings including living with their families and in community-based settings run by a number of organizations, both statutory bodies and in the private and voluntary sector. Some of these units are set up to deal specifically with challenging behaviour and therefore are more likely to have the appropriate staff and resources to work with this client group. Many people with intellectual disabilities and challenging behaviour are often placed in residential schools as children at great financial and emotional cost. In a study by Pilling et al. [17] the researchers found that lack of support, or inappropriate support for the family and child at home, was a major factor in the child being placed in a residential school.

Difficulties can arise when the person with challenging behaviour accesses a number of different environments, for example home, school and respite care; getting a consensus of opinion about the causes of and the ways to treat the challenging behaviour can be difficult.

Treatments for challenging behaviours are usually multi-modal and non-aversive, incorporating medication (where appropriate), behavioural psychotherapies and environmental manipulations with any treatment regime being executed only after a detailed assessment of the behaviour as described above. By far the major body of knowledge in the assessment and treatment of challenging behaviours comes from the arena of applied behaviour analysis and in particular operant conditioning. Behavioural assessment of challenging behaviours has concentrated on finding the function(s), or purpose, that challenging behaviour(s) serve for the individual [11] while behavioural treatments have focused on the reduction of challenging behaviours by increasing the competencies of the individual, particularly in regard to the person's expressive communication. Engaging with the individual and the members of their system is central to ensuring optimal treatment.

Support is very important and it needs to be sensitive and appropriate not just to the individual's needs but also to the family. Collaborative and integrated multidisciplinary, multi-agency working can maximize the value of support.

Positive behaviour support

Positive behaviour support (PBS) is a combined behavioural analysis and person centred approach to working with challenging behaviour. The aim of PBS is to replace difficult behaviour with functionally equivalent behaviours while at the same time looking at and changing environmental and social factors that influence the behaviour or maintain it. PBS signified a move away from punitive techniques for managing behaviour towards positive, non-aversive techniques (such as those put forward by Donnellan, LaVigna et al. [18]) while increasing communication and other skills for the client. A good PBS plan would include:

- Descriptions of replacement behaviours and how these should be implemented.

- Teaching functionally equivalent behaviours and communication and when and how these will be taught.

- The manipulation of setting events that lead to the person displaying challenging behaviour.

- The manipulation of antecedents and consequences to behaviour.

- How and when appropriate behaviour should be rewarded or reinforced.

Case vignette 9.4

John engages in aggressive behaviours in demand situations (when on task in the classroom). A functional assessment has revealed that this behaviour is used to avoid completing tasks. A programme to teach John how to escape from situations appropriately using a card to request a 'break' has been implemented and the appropriate behaviour has been reinforced.

Role of improving quality of life for people with intellectual disabilities and carers

Improving the quality of life for the individual with person centred planning and empowering the individual to have more control over their lives is likely to result in more satisfying lives and simultaneously eliminate some of the causes of challenging behaviour.

Management of chronic challenging behaviour

By definition chronic challenging behaviour will have been continuing for a long time, often years. It is likely that many intensive interventions in the past have failed. The perpetuating factors whether by the nature of the individual or of their network of support are likely to be deeply entrenched. The major challenges when the behaviour is chronic are to maintain therapeutic optimism and to maintain a clear and consistent strategy. It is likely that the network of support will have tried many strategies and people are likely to have been requested to fill in behaviour monitoring charts numerous times, so suggestions are often met with the refrain that they have tried that before and degrees of anger can be expected when family and carers are asked to complete 'yet more charts'. Many teams operate with limited resources and cannot provide the intensive support that might make a difference. This can contribute to carers feeling let down and professionals feeling powerless and undervalued. Being able to acknowledge our limitations can help. It is important to communicate these limitations to managers and commissioners. Despite this, surprising successes can be achieved:

Case vignette 9.5

The challenging behaviour team had been working with Robert and his carers in a specialist residential home for people with autism for some years. Robert

---

continued to self-injure on and off, as he had for many years, and the team concluded that he needed to move to a new home with a consistent person centred approach. Robert moved to his own flat with support and the behaviour ceased.

Medication for challenging behaviour

Challenging behaviour is an attribution given to a social construction, with no consistent relationship with any clinical condition believed to consistently respond to pharmaceutical intervention. To treat empirically solely with medication and without a rationale may be effective in reducing the frequency of the unwanted behaviour but is the antithesis of modern management of challenging behaviour: 'generalized suppression of behaviour can be acquainted with clinical desperation, and is only one small advance on physical restraint' [19].

Brylewski and Duggan's [20] Cochrane review of antipsychotic medication for challenging behaviour confirmed that there is not clear support for drug treatment. The NACHBID study similarly suggests the same conclusion [21]. Deb and colleagues [22] have produced a useful guide to using psychotropic medication. Whereas indiscriminate use of sedative medication may prevent the person from communicating their needs, appropriately targeted medication given to treat an underlying condition may result in the elimination of the challenging behaviour.

Treatment as experiment is true for medication too

All treatments are experiments that may or may not work. Awareness of the experimental nature of treatment helps the clinician to think of baseline measures and measures of treatment response, and to consult with the individual and their network about what degree of response might justify ongoing treatment (see also Chapter 14 on pharmacological interventions).

Specialist challenging behaviour services

Challenging behaviour brought to the attention of health or social care services can often be readily resolved. More severe and enduring challenging behaviour can exhaust the resources of primary care and community intellectual disability teams, who struggle to concentrate resources on the needs of a small number of severe cases while meeting the needs of the rest of the caseload.

Many of the skills of managing challenging behaviour are not unique to one professional discipline and many carers show impressive understanding and skills. A nurse can be just as much of an expert in functional analysis as a psychologist. The best way forward is to utilize the skills of a multidisciplinary team working in collaboration.

One of the disadvantages of specialist teams to address challenging behaviour is that they can be seen to be imposing their expertise on a demoralized and overburdened system. The challenge for specialist services is to transfer expertise and skills to the individual's immediate network, so that the network no longer requires the specialist input. There is a risk that when the network fails to retain this information, the specialists blame the network, rather than acknowledge their continuing role in maintaining the knowledge and skills in the community.

Multi-agency and interagency working

Much of the life of a person with an intellectual disability is controlled by others. In the case of children the control is usually mainly with the parents. For intellectually disabled adults, then, carers and social services, who often control funding for accommodation and day care, have far greater significance. Longer lasting and more effective solutions can be achieved with good communication and productive working relationships between the different components of the system.

A hundred years ago people with intellectual disabilities and their carers often lived in institutions cut off from wider society. The risk of continuing this isolationist mentality persists even now most of these people live in the community. Facilitating access to public facilities and to generic services is an important component in improving quality of life and quality of care for people with intellectual disabilities whether or not there is challenging behaviour. Educating others about resources and strengths within the intellectual disability community improves integration.

In-patient

Behaviours that result in admission to hospital are likely to qualify for conceptualization as challenging behaviour. The ward provides an environment where professionals can observe an individual's actions and conduct behavioural experiments to test hypotheses about the meaning and role of the behaviour. Removing the individual from their original environment may eliminate an undesirable behaviour because the circumstances that perpetuate it have been removed. Without understanding the underlying needs the behaviour is likely to re-emerge.

9.6 Conclusion

Challenging behaviour thinking encapsulates much of intellectual disabilities think-ing; the holistic consideration of physical, psychological and social and political aspects within a person centred and non-judgemental framework. A systematic approach to challenging behaviour has the potential to improve the care and the quality of life for the people involved. The concept of challenging behaviour confronts the moral attributions traditionally applied to people with intellectual disabilities. It counters the perverse predilection for punitive 'treatments', and inspires optimism that solutions can be found which enrich the life of the individual and those around them.

References

1. Emerson, E. (2001) *Challenging Behaviour: Analysis and Intervention in People with Severe Intellectual Disabilities*, 2nd edn, Cambridge University Press, Cambridge, p. 3.
2. Report of a Committee set up by the Mental Health Foundation (1997) Don't Forget Us – Children with Learning Disabilities and Severe Challenging Behaviour, The Mental Health Foundation, London, p. 12.
3. Clements, J. and Zarkowska, E. (2000) *Behavioural Concerns and Autistic Spectrum Disorders*, Jessica Kingsley Publishers, London.
4. Emerson, E., Kiernan, C., Alborz, A. *et al.* (2001) The prevalence of challenging behaviors: a total population study. *Research in Developmental Disabilities*, **22** (1), 77–93.
5. Qureshi, H. and Alborz, A. (1992) The epidemiology of challenging behaviour. *Mental Handicap Research*, **5**, 130–145.
6. Emerson, E. and Bromley, J. (1995) The form and function of challenging behaviours. *Journal of Intellectual Disability Research*, **39**, 388–398.
7. Baum S. and Lynggaard H. (eds) (2006) *Intellectual Disabilities: A Systemic Approach*, Karnac, London.
8. Department of Health (1993) Services for People with Learning Disabilities and Challenging Behaviour or Mental Health Needs, The 'Mansell Report', HMSO, London.
9. Royal College of Psychiatrists (2001) *Diagnostic Criteria for Psychiatric Disorders for Use with Adults with Learning Disabilities/Mental Retardation*, Gaskell, London.
10. Ball, T., Bush, A. and Emerson, E. (2004) *Challenging Behaviours: Psychological Interventions for Severely Challenging Behaviours Shown by People with Learning Disabilities. Clinical Practice Guidelines*, British Psychological Society, Leicester.
11. O'Neill, R.E., Horner, R.H., Albin, R.W. *et al.* (1997) *Functional Assessment and Program Development for Problem Behavior – A Practical Handbook*, 2nd edn, Brooks/Cole Publishing Company, Pacific Grove.
12. Zarkowska, E. and Clements, J. (1994) *Problem Behaviour and People with Severe Learning Disabilities (The STAR Approach)*, Chapman and Hall, London.
13. Durand, V.M. and Crimmins, D.B. (1992) *The Motivation Assessment Scale Administration Guide*, Monaco & Associates, Topeka.

14. Matson, J.L. and Vollmer, T. (1995) *Questions About Behavioral Function (QABF)*, Disability Consultants, LLC, Baton Rouge.

15. O'Brien, G., Pearson, J., Berney, T. and Barnard, L. (2001) Measuring behaviour in developmental disability: a review of existing schedules. *Developmental Medicine and Child Neurology*, **43** (Suppl 87), 1–72.

16. Department of Health (Mansell) (2007) *Services for People with Learning Disabilities and Challenging Behaviour or Mental Health Needs*, Department of Health, London.

17. Pilling, N., McGill, P. and Cooper, V. (2007) Characteristics and experiences of children and young people with severe intellectual disabilities and challenging behaviour attending 52-week residential special schools. *Journal of Intellectual Disability Research*, **51** (Part 3), 184–196.

18. Donnellan, A.M., LaVigna, G.W., Negri-Shoultz, N. and Fassbender, L.L. (1988) *Progress without Punishment – Effective Approaches for Learners with Behavior Problems*, Teachers College Press, New York.

19. Werry J. (1988) in *Psychopharmacology of the Developmental Disabilities* (eds M.G. Aman and N.N. Singh), Springer-Verlag, New York.

20. Brylewski, J. and Duggan, L. (2004) Antipsychotic medication for challenging behaviour in people with learning disability. *Cochrane Database of Systematic Reviews* [online] 3 (Art. No.: CD000377).

21. Tyrer, P. (2008) Risperidone, haloperidol, and placebo in the treatment of aggressive challenging behaviour in patients with intellectual disability: a randomised controlled trial. *Lancet*, **371**, 57–63.

22. Deb, S., Clarke, D. and Unwin, G. (2006) *Using Medication to Manage Behaviour Problems Among Adults with a Learning Disability*, Royal College of Psychiatrists, London.

Further reading

Banks, R. and Bush, A. (eds) (2007) *Challenging Behaviour: A Unified Approach*, Gaskell, London.

Sturmey, P. (1996) *Functional Analysis in Clinical Psychology*, John Wiley & Sons, Ltd, Chichester.

Clements, J. and Martin, N. (2002) *Assessing Behaviors Regarded as Problematic for People with Developmental Disabilities*, Jessica Kingsley Publishers, London.

10 Interaction between Mental and Physical Health

Michael Kerr[1] and Basil Cardoza[2]
[1]*Welsh Centre for Learning Disabilities, Cardiff, UK*
[2]*ABM University NHS Trust, Cardiff, UK*

10.1 Introduction

People with intellectual disabilities have increased and characteristic health needs. This is due to morbidities associated with specific aetiologies of the disability and also deterioration of physical conditions, which often go unreported. Following deinstitutionalization in the late 1980s and early 1990s, the prevalence rates of conditions usually associated with older age groups in the general population, like cancer and ischaemic heart disease, may be increasing.

To understand fully the interaction between physical and mental illness in people with intellectual disabilities, we need to consider several factors, which include:

- any underlying physical disability

- level of intellectual impairment

- premorbid personality

- previous experience of ill health

- interpersonal relationships

Intellectual Disability Psychiatry: a practical handbook   Angela Hassiotis, Diana Andrea Barron and Ian Hall (eds)
© 2009 John Wiley & Sons, Ltd

- perceived threat of illness

- physical treatment required.

The importance of this interface is highlighted by the high levels of morbidity and psychosocial neglect experienced by this population. Most illnesses may require a period of adjustment and re-evaluation of lifestyle. Using a biopsychosocial framework that accounts for the underlying influences on the clinical presentation, will help understand the individual and nature of the influences on health.

10.2 Biopsychosocial influences

An individual's genotype can determine not only their physical characteristics (phenotype), but also their behavioural characteristics (behavioural phenotype). This includes the development of either a physical disease or a psychiatric disorder. For example, individuals with intellectual disability and fragile X syndrome are predisposed to develop attention deficit hyperactivity disorder (ADHD) and complex partial epilepsy [1]. Self-injurious behaviours can be more frequent in Prader-Willi, Cornelia de Lange, Lesch Nyhan and Smith Magenis syndromes. Up to 30% of individuals with Prader-Willi syndrome, inherited by uniparental disomy, may develop a psychotic illness [2].

Similarly psychological and social factors can influence the expression of biological predispositions and vice-versa. The development of Alzheimer's disease will have significant psychosocial consequences, especially in those predisposed, like people with Down's syndrome. Nevertheless, people with intellectual disabilities also commonly present with a more complex interaction between biopsychosocial factors and their physical and mental health. For example, sexual abuse is more common in people with intellectual disabilities and may lead to physical and psychological trauma, which in turn may lead to behaviours that perpetuate the cycle of abuse [3].

Individual characteristics play an important role in shaping illness response. They influence how an illness is perceived and the patient's coping style. The coping strategies and defence mechanisms that help the general population cope constructively with illness may be less apparent in people with intellectual disabilities. A less obvious influence is the increased risk of physical and psychiatric morbidity and mortality, seen in the lower socio-economic classes and often in people with intellectual disabilities [4].

10.3 Physical morbidity

The general health status of people with intellectual disabilities is poor. There are reports of increased levels of unrecognized or inadequately managed physical morbidity in this group, both in institutions and in the community (see Table 10.1). Beange *et al.* [5] found that a person with intellectual disability had, on average, more medical conditions than a non-disabled person, with specialist care required in up to 74%. Sensory impairments, epilepsy and thyroid disease were considerably more common than in the general population.

The life expectancy of people with intellectual disabilities is significantly reduced, compared to the non-disabled population [6]. Their overall life expectancy of 68.7 years is significantly less than the general population and the reduction in life span is directly proportional to the level of disability [7]. A genetic aetiology, poor mobility and inability to feed themselves are further risk factors for premature death. For this reason *Valuing People 2001* suggested all people with intellectual disabilities would have a health action plan by June 2005.

Patients with intellectual disabilities are believed to have many untreated medical conditions, low levels of health promotion and preventative care. Several barriers to health care have been identified including mobility problems, challenging behaviour, communication difficulties, general practitioners' lack of specialist knowledge and the additional resources required. Health promotion, health screening, education of general practitioners and improving carer knowledge of health issues have all been suggested as methods of improving physical health in people with intellectual disabilities. The report of the independent inquiry into access to health care for people with learning disabilities, [8] led by Sir Jonathan Michael, was prompted by the Mencap Report *Death by Indifference*, which highlighted many of these issues, and aimed to identify the action needed to ensure adults and children with learning disabilities receive appropriate treatment in acute and primary health care in England. (see Table 10.2). The

Table 10.1 Frequencies of physical disorder in people with intellectual disability

Hearing impairments	10–28%
Vision impairments	10–44%
Obesity	9.8–44%
Dental disease	<20–29%
Epilepsy	14–44%
Incontinence	13–49.3%
Respiratory disease	43–75%

Table 10.2   Michael report recommendations

RECOMMENDATION 1: Those with responsibility for the provision and regulation of undergraduate and postgraduate clinical training, must ensure that curricula include mandatory training in learning disabilities. It should be competence-based and involve people with learning disabilities and their carers in providing training.

RECOMMENDATION 2: All healthcare organisations, including the Department of Health should ensure that they collect the data and information necessary to allow people with learning disability to be identified by the health service and their pathways of care tracked.

RECOMMENDATION 3: Family and other carers should be involved as a matter of course as partners in the provision of treatment and care, unless good reason is given, and Trust Boards should ensure that reasonable adjustments are made to enable them to do this effectively. This will include the provision of information, but may also involve practical support and service co-ordination.

RECOMMENDATION 4: Primary care trusts should identify and assess the needs of people with learning disabilities and their carers as part of their Joint Strategic Needs Assessment. They should consult with their Local Strategic Partnership, their Learning Disability Partnership Boards and relevant voluntary user-led learning disability organisations and use the information to inform the development of Local Area Agreements.

RECOMMENDATION 5: To raise awareness in the health service of the risk of premature avoidable death, and to promote sustainable good practice in local assessment, management and evaluation of services, the Department of Health should establish a learning disabilities Public Health Observatory. This should be supplemented by a time-limited Confidential Inquiry into premature deaths in people with learning disabilities to provide evidence for clinical and professional staff of the extent of the problem and guidance on prevention.

RECOMMENDATION 6: The Department of Health should immediately amend Core Standards for Better Health, to include an explicit reference to the requirement to make 'reasonable adjustments' to the provision and delivery of services for vulnerable groups, in accordance with the disability equality legislation. The framework that is planned to replace these core standards in 2010 should also include a specific reference to this requirement.

RECOMMENDATION 7: Inspectors and regulators of the health service should develop and extend their monitoring of the standard of general health services provided for people with learning disabilities, in both the hospital sector and in the community where primary care providers are located. The aim is to support appropriate, reasonable adjustments to general health services for adults and children with learning disabilities and their families and to ensure compliance with and enforcement of all aspects of the Disability Discrimination Act. Healthcare regulators and inspectors (and the Care Quality Commission, once established) should strengthen their work in partnership with each other and with the Commission for Equality and Human Rights, the National Patient Safety Agency and Office for Disability Issues).

Table 10.2   (*continued*)

RECOMMENDATION 8: The Department of Health should direct primary care trusts (PCTs) to secure general health services that make 'reasonable adjustments' for people with learning disabilities through a Directed Enhanced Service. In particular, the Department should direct PCTs to commission enhanced primary care services which include regular health checks provided by General Practitioner (GP) practices and improve data, communication and cross-boundary partnership working. This should include liaison staff who work with primary care services to improve the overall quality of health care for people with learning disabilities across the spectrum of care.

RECOMMENDATION 9: Section 242 of the National Health Service Act 2006 requires National Health Service (NHS) bodies to involve and consult patients and the public in the planning and development of services, and in decisions affecting the operation of services. All Trust Boards should ensure that the views and interests of people with learning disabilities and their carers are included.

RECOMMENDATION 10: All Trust Boards should demonstrate in routine public reports that they have effective systems in place to deliver effective, 'reasonably adjusted' health services for those people who happen to have a learning disability. This 'adjustment' should include arrangements to provide advocacy for all those who need it, and arrangements to secure effective representation on Patient Advice and Liaison Services (PALS) from all client groups including people with learning disabilities

report found evidence of both good practice, and 'examples of discrimination, abuse and neglect across the range of health services' and provided recommendations to help address these inequalities (see Chapter 16).

Structured health checks in primary care can identify clinically significant previously unrecognized morbidity among adults with intellectual disabilities and an annual health check is justifiable in this population. Felce *et al.* [9] confirmed previous findings that health needs can be identified among adults with an intellectual disability who may fail to report symptoms because of restricted communication or social or other impairments, and appropriate health promotion undertaken, through the use of structured health checks. The study also concluded that health checking is an effective intervention for identifying remedial general health problems among people with intellectual disabilities and that annual health checking was justifiable.

Good practice example

The 'Welsh Health Check for adults with an intellectual disability and on the social register' introduced in Wales entitles every person with an intellectual disability to have an annual medical review along with appropriate investigations. This comprises a comprehensive screening process including immunization status, cervical and breast screening, systems enquiry, presence of epilepsy and behavioural disorders, followed by a complete physical examination.

10.4 Interaction between physical and mental health

A wide range of psychiatric diagnoses have been described following a physical illness in the general population, the commonest of which are listed in Table 10.3. Adjustment disorder is probably the most common psychological reaction that satisfies the criteria for a psychiatric diagnosis. Anxiety may present as a range of disorders, including generalized anxiety disorder, panic disorder and phobia, all of which can be seen after a physical illness. Ryan, [10] in a major study of adults with intellectual disabilities, showed that sexual abuse by multiple perpetrators was the most common abuse suffered, followed by physical trauma and life threatening neglect. It also showed that people with intellectual disabilities developed post-traumatic stress disorder at a rate comparable to the general population, following exposure to trauma. Depressive disorders are common following a physical illness (e.g. neurological, endocrine and collagen disorders, infections and malignant disease).

Psychiatric disorders can have significant influence on physical health in a person with intellectual disability. Depression and psychotic disorders may predispose to poor compliance with medication, and diets and chronic psychiatric illnesses are known to be associated with poor physical health and increased morbidity.

Suicide is rarely reported in people with intellectual disabilities; this may be due to reluctance on behalf of the authorities to designate sudden death as suicide. While in the general population, women were more likely to attempt suicide than men,

Table 10.3 Psychiatric diagnosis following physical illness

Mental health diagnosis	Associated physical health diagnoses
Depressive and adjustment disorders	Neurological disorders (stroke, head injury, Parkinson's disease)
	Endocrine disorders (thyroid and parathyroid disorders, Cushing's syndrome)
	Malignancy (cerebral tumours, non-metastatic effects of other tumours)
	Infections (encephalitis, pneumonia, urinary tract infection)
Anxiety disorders	Myocardial infarction
Psychotic disorders	Space occupying brain lesion, epilepsy, Parkinson's disease, dementia
Sexual dysfunction	Stroke, diabetes, multiple sclerosis
Eating disorders	Diabetes

the opposite is true in the intellectually impaired. The majority seem to have a mild disability or have a borderline IQ. Younger age group, chronic health problems and a physical disability are also considered to be risk factors.

Sensory impairment

Higher rates of vision and hearing impairments have been reported in people with intellectual disabilities. This problem is often exacerbated by poor detection rates, more so in the severely disabled and individuals with communication difficulties. [5, 11] Carers often fail to identify hearing and visual impairments. People with intellectual disabilities will benefit from early recognition and treatment of sensory impairments, which will further reduce handicap and promote social acceptance.

The prevalence of hearing impairment ranges from 10 to 28% [5, 12] and might occur secondary to middle ear infections, impacted ear wax or with old age. People with fragile X and Noonan syndromes have a higher prevalence of hearing loss secondary to otitis media and perforated tympanum. High prevalence of both conductive and sensori-neural hearing loss is seen in Down's syndrome and impaired hearing may play a role in decline of social and cognitive functioning.

A wide range of visual impairments occur in people with intellectual disabilities, including refractive errors, strabismus and internal ocular disorders. People with Prader-Willi and Noonan syndromes are prone to visual problems. People with severe or profound intellectual disabilities are also more likely to have visual impairments, mostly due to optic nerve or cortical dysfunction. Ocular abnormalities involving almost all structures of the eye are especially common in Down's syndrome. Refractive errors, keratoconus, strabismus, cataracts, nystagmus and blepharitis have all been reported.

Deaf people depend on gestures and body language to communicate. Thus, behaviour which may appear overly animated may reflect a style of communication rather than an agitated state. Hearing and visual impairments can predispose to organic hallucinosis. Delusional elaboration of hallucinations may occur with insight often preserved. The overall prevalence of mental illness among deaf people is at least as high as in the population at large. Deaf people who are psychotic can display disorders of thought form and/or thought content. Thought form disorders are more difficult to diagnose and can include loose associations, flight of ideas, incoherence, tangentiality and fragmentation. One must consider that the ability to determine a thought disturbance can be compounded by a limited language system. Deaf people (including those with congenital deafness) experiencing psychosis may experience auditory hallucinations. People with intellectual disabilities are sometimes known to have dual sensory impairment (visual and hearing), which can pose a significant challenge for both carers and the treating psychiatrist.

Case vignette 10.1

Ms C is a 68-year-old woman with a moderate intellectual impairment, severe challenging behaviours, near total blindness and significant deafness. She lost her vision due to self-injurious behaviours, which resulted in enucleation of both eyes. Prior to the onset of her sensory impairments, she had a diagnosis of paranoid schizophrenia. She communicates to a very limited extent with her carers by touch, which serves her basic needs. At times of relapse of challenging behaviours, it can be extremely difficult to conduct an appropriate mental state examination. It was felt by carers that she often had paranoid ideas regarding other residents she lived with. She also had difficulties with sleep and her diurnal rhythm was altered due to lack of external cues.

Obesity

Studies on obesity in people with intellectual disabilities need to be treated with caution, due to several factors. Standards used in the general population may not be appropriate due to differences in body size and growth rate. There is also variation in the tools used to measure obesity, with some studies relying on height and weight tables and others measuring tricep skinfold thickness. Despite this, obesity is considered to be more prevalent in people with intellectual disabilities, more so in females [13]. Living in the community, especially in family homes, and having mild or moderate intellectual disabilities have also been suggested as risk factors, though disputed. Obesity is also associated with Prader-Willi, Down's, Carpenter and Cohen syndromes.

In Down's syndrome, being overweight or obese is a particular health problem due to reduced physical activity, poor diet control, lower basal metabolic rate and associated medical problems like hypothyroidism. There is an earlier decline in weight with age, as compared to the general population, which may be due to an early ageing process.

Obesity is also a problem in people with severe mental illness. Metabolic diseases, including obesity, are likely to contribute to increased mortality in this population. Whether mental illness in itself is an independent risk factor for the development of obesity and other components of the metabolic syndrome, or whether metabolic dysfunction is simply secondary to lifestyle remains unclear. Iatrogenic causes of obesity are also likely to be important, as weight gain may be caused by atypical antipsychotic drugs and some anti-epileptic drugs.

Obesity has potentially far reaching physical implications, and hence it is important to target people with intellectual disabilities at risk. Behavioural strategies with carer involvement, increasing physical activity and dietary control are all useful in reducing weight.

Underweight

Low weight in people with intellectual disabilities is usually related to feeding difficulties, placing the individual at risk for malnutrition. People with more severe intellectual disabilities are more at risk due to a soft diet, food regurgitation, immobility and carer reliance. Having a neurological impairment or cerebral palsy is considered a risk factor for being underweight. Kennedy *et al.* [14] showed that people with intellectual disabilities had normal protein intake, but their intake of fat and carbohydrates were reduced due to swallowing difficulties.

Dental health

There is an increased prevalence of poor oral hygiene, gum disease, dental caries and loss of teeth in people with intellectual disabilities, which does not seem to be related to their level of physical ability or manual dexterity. Previous studies have indicated that they seem to receive less restorative care, but this trend seems to be improving. Dental abnormalities are also associated with Angelman's and fragile X syndromes due to their particular phenotypes.

Anticholinergic drugs and several antipsychotic drugs may cause a dry mouth, which has a significant impact on oral health and increases the risk of dental caries, periodontal disease and oral infections like candidiasis. This could present as difficulty with speech, chewing, swallowing and poor denture tolerance. Dyskinesia and dystonia are distressing side effects of antipsychotic drugs, characterized by abnormal jaw and/or tongue movements. Certain anti-epileptic drugs like phenytoin are known to cause periodontal disease like gingivitis.

Incontinence

Rates of incontinence in people with intellectual disabilities vary from 13% to almost 50% depending on their age, with higher prevalence rates in those aged above 65 years, due to their worsening sensory impairment and mobility. This can cause considerable difficulties for individuals and carers. Incontinence may herald the onset of an infection, or occur as a challenging behaviour, a method of communication or as learnt behaviour.

Epilepsy

Epilepsy rates in people with intellectual disabilities are much higher than in the general population. Various studies have found prevalence rates of 14–44% [15], 16.1% [16] and 18% [17]. There is a strong association between prevalence of epilepsy and severity of disability, the highest being reported in institutionalized patients. Many epilepsy syndromes which are severe and frequently associated with significant intellectual disabilities are known as epileptic encephalopathies and the intellectual impairment is related to a combination of the underlying disorder, the frequency of seizures, and abnormal electroencephalogram (EEG) activity.

A potential and important cause of intellectual disability may be the aetiology of the epilepsy syndrome itself. This may occur as part of a chromosomal disorder (e.g. Down's syndrome, Ring chromosome 20), a genetic syndrome (e.g. Prader-Willi syndrome, Rett syndrome), or as a consequence of early brain injury. Epilepsy is also particularly associated with Lennox-Gastaut, Landau-Kleffener, West, Angelman's and Wolf-Hirschhorn syndromes. Treatment resistant epilepsy and mild to severe intellectual disabilities are characteristic features of most neurocutaneous syndromes like tuberous sclerosis.

Epilepsy seems to present as more complex in this group and is often treatment resistant. Some studies have reported generalized tonic-clonic seizures as the most common. Complex partial seizures seem to be the most common in people with intellectual disabilities and autism. People with intellectual disabilities and epilepsy also seem to have higher rates of psychogenic non-epileptic seizures.

There is an increased prevalence of psychiatric disorder in people with intellectual disabilities and epilepsy. Depression and psychoses were found to be more common in those with no seizures in the preceding three months, compared to patients who had at least one seizure in the same period. Rates of psychosis were also higher in those with milder disability and epilepsy, whereas depression rates were higher in those with severe disability. Some studies on children with and without intellectual disabilities have shown no significant differences in the frequency of behavioural disturbances, while others have reported hyperactivity, antisocial behaviour and schizophrenia-like psychosis in children with intellectual disabilities, especially in association with temporal lobe epilepsy.

Epilepsy and its treatment can have a profound effect on individuals with intellectual disabilities. This impact on physical health, psychological health and mortality has, in turn, a further impact on the families and carers for these individuals [18]. Anti-epileptic drugs of proven efficacy in the general population are also effective in refractory epilepsy in people with intellectual disabilities [19]. Higher response rates have been reported in focal and multifocal epilepsy as compared to symptomatic generalized epilepsy/Lennox Gastaut syndrome. Adverse reactions to anti-epileptic drugs are seen in more than a third of these patients, somnolence and ataxia the most common. Vigabatrine has been shown to precipitate psychotic and affective symptoms. Skin drug reactions are significantly less often seen in people with intellectual disabilities and epilepsy, and are more common in females than males. A systematic review on non-pharmacological interventions for epilepsy in people with intellectual disabilities found no randomized controlled studies in this population [20].

Case vignette 10.2

Mr H is a 29 year old man with moderate intellectual disability, Autistic Spectrum disorder (ASD), idiopathic generalized epilepsy, and significant self-injurious and challenging behaviours. He presented with generalized tonic-clonic and complex partial seizures, which have been resistant to treatment, and is currently on two anti-epileptic drugs. Previously, he was on several other anti-epileptic drugs to which he showed only partial response. The treatment options have also been limited because of his susceptibility to side effects of medication. His seizures have also led to confusional states, injuries and a decline in his community activities.

Respiratory disease

Mortality rates in people with intellectual disabilities due to respiratory disease range from 43 to 75%, compared to 8% in the general population. The more severely disabled have higher rates and seem to be more likely to die from an infectious respiratory disease. The risk is also increased by immobility, physical disabilities, food aspiration problems and being underweight. Individuals with Down's syndrome tend to have a particular problem with recurrent chest infections, but the less disabled in this group are more likely to die from respiratory infections.

The diagnosis of depression may be difficult in patients with chronic respiratory disease, due to the overlap of depressive and pulmonary symptoms like fatigue, weight loss, anorexia and loss of interest.

Cardiovascular disease

Due to their increased risk of obesity, people with intellectual disabilities are also at higher risk of heart disease, myocardial infarction and metabolic syndromes. People with Down's syndrome are at particular risk because of the presence of congenital heart problems and their propensity to premature ageing.

A significant proportion of survivors of myocardial infarction suffer from major depressive illness, although it is important to differentiate between those whose depression was precipitated by the infarction and those who were psychologically unwell prior to the infarction.

Other medical disorders

Relatively common medical disorders are often missed in people with intellectual disabilities, especially when associated with communication difficulties and should be considered when presenting with challenging behaviours. They include:

1. Adverse reactions secondary to medication – for example akathisia secondary to antipsychotic drugs, headache and diplopia secondary to anti-epileptic drugs, toxicity secondary to lithium.
2. Unrecognized pain due to trauma, dental disease, constipation, musculoskeletal disease, reflux oesophagitis, etc.
3. Delirium is characterized by clouding of consciousness and impairment of cognition, with a reduced ability to focus, typically lasting for hours or days. The elderly and the severely intellectually disabled are more at risk. People with intellectual disabilities, especially of the severe type, are also more likely to have unrecognized delirium which may lead to delays in treatment. Delirium in the intellectual disability population usually indicates the presence of underlying disease and includes infection (respiratory tract, urinary tract and ear), faecal impaction, urinary retention, electrolyte disturbances, dehydration and medications (anti-epileptics, antipsychotics, anticholinergics, etc.).

Case vignette 10.3

Ms W is a 32-year-old woman with moderate to severe intellectual disability, very limited communication, challenging behaviours and a history of recurrent urinary tract infections. She presents with episodes resembling delirium, which require a prompt physical examination to exclude an organic cause. Due to her pre-existing cognitive impairment and limited communication, it was often difficult to conclude as to the presence or absence of a delirium. More often than not, it has been found that when delirium was present, the aetiology was a relapse of her urinary tract infection.

Cancer

Prior to deinstitutionalization, cancer was not of significant concern in people with intellectual disabilities, accounting for about 15% of deaths in this population. With the increase in life expectancy, especially in the more severely disabled, prevalence of cancer may be increasing. Gastrointestinal cancers are more common, and breast and prostate cancers are less common, compared to the general population. Increased levels of independence, greater access and choice, especially in people with milder disabilities, may lead to higher levels of smoking and use of alcohol, putting them at risk.

Many psychiatric disorders may occur in patients with cancer including adjustment disorder, delirium, anxiety disorders and depression.

Autistic spectrum disorders

Autistic spectrum disorders are discussed in further detail elsewhere (Chapter 7) Most cases of autism do not have a known aetiology, however, between 10 and 30% of cases of ASDs are associated with known syndromes.

About a third of individuals with ASD experience seizures, the prevalence varying with the level of disability. As individuals with autism may have communication difficulties, seizures may go unrecognized. Up to 20% of children with ASDs may have an abnormal EEG, with no history of seizures.

Tuberous sclerosis

Psychiatric and behavioural symptoms have been described in tuberous sclerosis, including hyperactivity, aggression, seizures, obsessive compulsive disorders, schizophrenia and depressive disorders. Autistic features occur in about 60% of patients and epidemiological studies have suggested a strong association between the two disorders. The degree of impairment and risk of autism are proportional to the location and number of cortical tumours, with a substantial increase when the tubers are located in the temporal area.

Cerebral palsy

ASD was found in almost a fifth of children with cerebral palsy and intellectual or physical disabilities, and strictly defined autism in about 9% in a Scandinavian study. A close association was found between intellectual disability, epilepsy and ASD in this group of children with neurodevelopmental disorders [21]. The rate of cerebral palsy was found to be higher in a group of autistic children in France, compared to the general population. Patients with cerebral palsy and autistic behaviours can be wrongly labelled as having challenging behaviours.

10.5 Conclusions

To gain a better understanding of the interface between physical and mental health, we need to consider the biological, psychological and social circumstances of the individual. People with intellectual disabilities experience multiple physical and psychiatric disorders and often one predisposes to the other. It is essential to include a detailed physical assessment and consider any possible impact this might have on presenting behaviours and symptoms.

References

1. Hagerman R.J. and Cronister A. (eds) (1996) *Fragile X Syndrome: Diagnosis, Treatment and Research*, 2nd edn, The John Hopkins University Press, Baltimore, London.
2. Boer, H., Holland, A., Whittington, J. *et al.* (2002) Psychotic illness in people with Prader-Willi syndrome due to chromosome 15 maternal uniparental disomy. *Lancet*, **359**, 135–136.
3. Sobsey, D. and Doe, T. (1991) Patterns of sexual abuse and assault. *Sexuality and Disability*, **9**, 243–259.
4. Emerson, E. (2003) Mothers of children and adolescents with intellectual disability: social and economic situation, mental health status and the self assessed social and psychological impact of the child's difficulties. *Journal of Intellectual Disability Research*, **47**, 385–399.
5. Beange, H., McElduff, A. and Baker, W. (1995) Medical disorders of adults with mental retardation: a population study. *American Journal of Mental Retardation*, **99**, 595–604.
6. Durvasula, S., Beange, H. and Baker, W. (2002) Mortality of people with intellectual disability in Northern Sydney. *Journal of Intellectual and Developmental Disability*, **27**, 255–264.
7. Bittles, A.H., Petterson, B.A., Sullivan, S.G. *et al.* (2002) The influence of intellectual disability on life expectancy. *Journals of Gerontology*, **57A**, 470–472.
8. Michael, J. (2008) *Report of the Independent Inquiry into Access to Healthcare for People with Learning Disabilities*, Mencap, London.
9. Felce, D., Baxter, H., Lowe, K. *et al.* (2008) The Impact of Repeated Health Checks for Adults with Intellectual Disabilties. *Journal of Applied Research in Intellectual Disabilities*, **21**, 585–596.
10. Ryan, R. (1994) Post-traumatic stress disorder in persons with developmental disabilities. *Community Mental Health Journal*, **30**, 45–53.
11. Evenhuis, H. (1995a) Medical aspects of ageing in a population with intellectual disability: I. Visual impairment. *Journal of Intellectual Disability Research*, **39**, 19–25.
12. Evenhuis, H. (1995b) Medical aspects of ageing in a population with intellectual disability: II. Hearing impairment. *Journal of Intellectual Disability Research*, **39**, 27–33.
13. Bell, A.J. and Bhate, M.S. (1992) Prevalence of overweight and obesity in Down's syndrome and other mentally handicapped adults living in the community. *Journal of Learning Disability Research*, **36**, 359–364.
14. Kennedy, M., McCombie, L., Dawes, P. *et al.* (1997) Nutritional support for patients with learning disability and nutrition/dysphagia disorders in community care. *Journal of Learning Disability Research*, **41**, 430–436.
15. Bowley, C. and Kerr, M. (2000) Epilepsy and intellectual disability. *Journal of Intellectual Disability Research*, **44**, 529–543.
16. Morgan, C.L., Baxter, H. and Kerr, M.P. (2003) Prevalence of epilepsy and associated health service utilization and mortality among patients with Intellectual Disability. *American Journal of Mental Retardation*, **108** (5), 293–300.

17. Matthews, T., Weston, N., Baxter, H. *et al.* (2008) A general practice-based prevalence study of epilepsy among adults with intellectual disabilities and of it's association with psychiatric disorder, behaviour disturbance and carer stress. *Journal of Intellectual Disability Research*, **52** (Pt 2), 163–173.
18. Kerr, M. and Bowley, C. (2001) Evidence-based prescribing in those with learning disability and epilepsy. *Epilepsia*, **42** (Suppl 1), 44–45.
19. Beavis, J., Kerr, M. and Marson, A.G. (2007) Pharmacological interventions for epilepsy in people with intellectual disabilities. *Cochrane Database of Systematic Reviews* 3 (Art. No.: CD005399). doi: 10.1002/14651858.CD005399.pub2.
20. Beavis, J., Kerr, M. and Marson, A.G. (2007) Non-pharmacological interventions for epilepsy in people with intellectual disabilities. *Cochrane Database of Systematic Reviews* 4 (Art. No.: CD005502). doi: 10.1002/14651858.CD005502.pub2
21. Gillberg, C. and Coleman, M. (1996) Autism and medical disorders: a review of the literature. *Developmental Medicine and Child Neurology*, **38**, 191–202.

Further reading

Fraser W. and Kerr M. (eds) (2003) *Seminars in the Psychiatry of Learning Disabilities*, 2nd edn, The Royal College of Psychiatrists, Gaskell.

Bouras N. and Holt G. (eds) (2007) *Psychiatric and Behavioural Disorders in Intellectual and Developmental Disabilities*, 2nd edn, Cambridge University Press.

Lloyd G. and Guthrie E. (eds) (2007) *Handbook of Liaison Psychiatry*, Cambridge University Press.

11 Mental Health of Older People

Andre Strydom[1] and Jennifer Torr[2]

[1]Department of Mental Health Sciences, University College London, UK
[2]Centre for Developmental Health Victoria, Monash University, Australia

11.1 Introduction

Older people with intellectual disabilities are a rapidly growing population as a result of increases in life expectancy from 20 years to more than 60 years over the last century combined with the ageing of people born during the baby boom. Consequently physical and mental disorders of ageing in older people with intellectual disabilities have become important issues in clinical practice and for service providers in meeting the increasing care needs of this group. There is no firm agreement as to what is meant by 'older people' with intellectual disabilities. The sixth decade is when age-related issues start to emerge. However, people with Down's syndrome may face significant age-related disorders in the fifth decade. As more people with intellectual disabilities are living into old age there is increasing focus on elderly people, aged 65 years plus.

11.2 Health and ageing of older adults with intellectual disabilities

People with intellectual disabilities are a heterogeneous group, with differential survival rates. In general 50% of people with intellectual disabilities die before the age of 50 years and the most common cause of death is respiratory failure [1]. Early mortality is associated with specific syndromes with serious congenital abnormalities

Intellectual Disability Psychiatry: a practical handbook   Angela Hassiotis, Diana Andrea Barron and Ian Hall (eds)
© 2009 John Wiley & Sons, Ltd

and/or metabolic or immune disorders, severe and profound intellectual disabilities, epilepsy, sensory impairments, immobility and limited self-care skills.

As a result of selective mortality, older people with intellectual disabilities tend to have milder intellectual disability and better health than the population with intellectual disabilities as a whole. Population studies have shown lower rates of smoking, alcohol consumption and illicit drug use than for the general population. However, people with intellectual disabilities often have poor nutrition, sedentary lifestyle and obesity. Other vascular risk such as hyperlipidaemia and hypertension may not be identified or well managed. Cardiovascular disease is a major cause of death although the risk may be less than for the general population [2]. However, most studies are conducted on the identified population with intellectual disabilities who are known to services. Little is known about the health of people with borderline/mild intellectual disabilities who may not be known to disability services. This hidden group could have higher rates of cigarette, alcohol and drug use and other lifestyle risk factors increasing the risk of age-related health problems.

Older people with intellectual disabilities have a range of other health problems, many of which remain unidentified or untreated. The prevalence of vision and hearing impairments is greater than for the general population [3]. Institutional and group care can result in higher rate of chronic infectious disease such as hepatitis B and Helicobacter pylori infections. The incidence of oesophageal [4] and gastric cancers [5] are higher than for the general population and may reflect undiagnosed and untreated gastro-oesophageal disease and gastric ulcers.

The musculoskeletal system is particularly prone to age-related change. Combinations of congenital joint abnormalities, connective tissue laxity, neurological motor impairments and lack of exercise and poor muscle strength can lead to the premature development of osteoarthritis. There are higher rates of osteoporosis. Falls are common in older people with intellectual disabilities and are associated with epilepsy, impaired vision and medications such as anticonvulsants and psychotropics. Falls and osteoporosis result in fractures to both long bones and vertebrae [6].

Sub-groups of older people with intellectual disabilities have specific age-related problems. For example people with cerebral palsy are at increased risk of earlier mortality due to motor impairments, epilepsy and aspiration pneumonia secondary to reflux and disorders of chewing and swallowing. Morbidity also increases with age with diminished muscle strength, increased spasticity, decreased mobility and balance, increased falls with a risk of fractures due to osteoporosis associated with long-term anticonvulsant and psychotropic medications, poor nutrition and limited weight bearing activities. Pain associated with spasticity and fractures may be overlooked because of communication impairments [7].

People with Down's syndrome have high rates and early onset of a number of age-related disorders including vision and hearing impairments, [3] osteoporosis [8] and arthritis [9] as well as Alzheimer's disease, [10] which will be discussed later.

Little is known about disorders of ageing in other genetic syndromes as the overall numbers of people with each syndrome reaching old age are small. What is apparent is that older people have many health problems secondary to chronic health problems specific to the genetic disorder; for example, few people with Prader Willi syndrome reach older age and those who do have a range of health problems secondary to obesity, higher risk of osteoporosis and fractures due to hypogonadism, hypotonia and low activity levels, sleep disorders and recurrent respiratory infections.

Health problems, pain and discomfort in older people with intellectual disabilities are easily overlooked resulting in individual suffering, increased morbidity and levels of disability, behavioural and functional change which could be mistaken for a behavioural or mental health problem and treated with psychotropic medications.

11.3 Psychosocial aspects of ageing

Older people with intellectual disabilities are often challenged by decline in health, pain and increased dependency. Cognitive decline may impact on a person's ability to cope and adapt. Even with a focus on person centred planning, the older person may not have much real control over their circumstances. Adaptation to the physical and cognitive changes of ageing may need to be mediated by others, who must first recognize the changes and the impact on the person's daily functioning before being able to facilitate choice and access to health and other services. For example in many jurisdictions people living in group homes are expected to work or attend day programmes even when unwell if care staff are not rostered during the day. There may be few options regarding retirement or there may be an expectation that retirement is not until 60 or 65 years. A day programme or employment that has become physically or cognitively too demanding can lead to resistive and aggressive behaviours. Rather than medication a person may actually require a change in their day programme, having opportunities to socialize with their peers, or being able to stay at home.

Older age is often a time of change and loss, including the separation from, or death of family, friends and carers. Decline in functioning may result in transitions in accommodation, which may affect some groups more than others. Older people with Down's syndrome are more likely to have major life events and change of accommodation, breach of pre-existing relationships, than their same age peers as a result of ill health and onset of dementia [11].

In many developed countries, parents of the current cohort of older people with intellectual disabilities were often encouraged to place their child into institutional care. As a cohort older people with intellectual disabilities are therefore more likely to have had institutional care since childhood and many may have no contact with their family. Deinstitutionalization is an ongoing process in many countries. Older people are often the last group to be moved from institutional to community care. This move might disrupt long-term social relationships and cause transitional stress as the person adapts to a new physical and social environment and changed daily routines.

When family relationships have been maintained, older people with intellectual disabilities may have ageing parents who face their own age-related issues. Ageing parents may no longer be able visit their son or daughter, or may no longer be able to continue to care for their older child who lives at home with them, due to their own problems or because of the increased care needs of their son or daughter. Sudden infirmity and death of a parent may result in unplanned emergency accommodation and a number of moves before settling into long-term accommodation.

Grief reactions may be unrecognized or the significance of the death minimized by family and care staff. People with intellectual disabilities may be excluded from the rites of passage and remembrance. Bereavement is often associated with anxiety, depression, adjustment disorder and behavioural change which may persist for longer than in the general population. Carers may find it difficult to provide emotional support for a variety of reasons and grief counselling (using a variety of methods including talking, drawing, looking at picture books and photographs) might be required.

11.4 Mental health of older people with intellectual disabilities

The prevalence of many mental health problems, including behaviour, anxiety and psychotic disorders, does not increase with age [12]. However, lifetime prevalence of affective disorder, in particular depression, increases with age. The diagnosis of mental illness in intellectual disabilities is covered in Chapters 5 and 6. As in the general population dementia is a common disorder of older age in people with intellectual disabilities and will be discussed later in this chapter.

Older people with intellectual disabilities may have undiagnosed mental illnesses and associated problem behaviours, or they may have been treated with psychotropic medication for many years without review. They are more likely to be taking antipsychotic and anticholinergic medications than their younger peers [13]. A detailed file review is important in identifying possible mental illnesses and original indications for treatments. Adverse effects of psychotropic medications are responsible for much morbidity. Extrapyramidal side effects impair mobility and swallowing, increasing risk of falls, aspiration pneumonia and death. Anticholinergic medications used to treat extrapyramidal side effects impair cognition or precipitate delirium. The sedating effects of many psychotropics impair functioning and increase risk of falls. Doses may need to adjusted downwards due to impairments in liver and renal functioning.

Case vignette 11.1

A 55-year-old man with mild intellectual disability, admitted to an institution in infancy, had been treated with typical antipsychotic depot medication at a high dose for decades for aggressive and destructive behaviours. He had marked extrapyramidal side effects. He had been at his current accommodation for only a few months and in that time his carers reported no particular behaviour problems. Detailed file review revealed recurrent episodes, lasting many months, characterized by 'giggling', loud talking and shouting, aggressive behaviour, property destruction including smashing windows, high activity levels including walking to the next town at night, and marked weight loss. There was no documentation suggestive of depressive episodes. It is likely that he has bipolar disorder and required treatment with a mood stabilizer and an atypical antipsychotic. He was also compliant with oral medications, and depot medication is probably not indicated.

Case vignette 11.2

Joan is a 60-year-old lady with mild intellectual disability, who lived with her elderly parents and had not previously accessed disability services. Her father had a prolonged illness over a few years and died six months prior to presentation. Joan had a history of poorly controlled diabetes, recurrent falls and recent onset of seizures. During her father's illness Joan had become tearful, irritable and withdrawn. Her family doctor treated her with an antidepressant, which was well tolerated and resulted in a significant improvement in mood. Following her father's death she became highly distressed, agitated and assaulted her frail elderly mother, who had a range of health problems and required community supports. The family doctor phoned the local mental health team and was advised to stop the antidepressant and commence a high dose of a sedating antipsychotic medication.

Joan's elderly mother had to deal with her own grief and poor health and could no longer continue to provide the lifetime of care to her daughter. Temporary crisis accommodation was found for Joan in another town, with a change in her primary health care provider. Joan now had to cope with the death of her father, separation from her mother as well as a major life transition. Her behaviour continued to escalate and the dose of the antipsychotic medication was increased. Behaviour charts documented that Joan was confused and disoriented but no longer aggressive. No adjustments were made to the dose of antipsychotic medication. Joan had a prolonged generalized seizure.

Over the following two weeks Joan became increasingly drowsy and by the time she was admitted to hospital was barely rousable. A CT scan of her brain revealed a massive subdural haematoma with mass effect. Following neurosurgery Joan regained consciousness but was completely dependent and required full nursing care.

Superficial psychiatric assessment, indiscriminate use of potent sedating medications, lack of follow-up and loss of continuity in-care all contributed to the unfortunate outcome.

11.5 Dementia

Dementia is an umbrella term for a group of brain disorders characterized by an acquired and often progressive syndrome of cognitive impairments, including decline in memory and other cognitive functions, severe enough to impair activities of daily living. The most common dementias are Alzheimer's disease and vascular dementia, which may occur together. Other dementias such as Lewy body dementia, dementia associated with Parkinson's disease and fronto-temporal dementia have also been described in people with intellectual disabilities.

Application of ICD-10 and DSM-IV standard diagnostic criteria for dementia may be difficult in individuals with intellectual disabilities because of difficulty in demonstrating decline in cognitive functioning given pre-existing cognitive deficits. The key to dementia diagnosis in adults with intellectual disabilities is a decline from an individual level of functioning [14]. Hence baseline cognitive assessments of adults with intellectual disabilities are recommended, especially for adults with Down's syndrome, who are at high risk of early onset Alzheimer's disease. However, this is generally not implemented by services.

ICD-10 criteria require evidence of a decline in both memory and thinking which is sufficient to impair personal activities of daily living. The impairment of memory typically affects the registration, storage and retrieval of new information, but previously learned and familiar material may also be lost, particularly in the later stages. In addition the ICD-10 requires a decline in emotional control and motivation or a change in social behaviour [15]. The diagnosis of 'dementia' is made when symptoms have been present for a minimum of six months and other causes, which are potentially treatable, have been ruled out. It is important to note that the neurodegenerative dementias generally progress gradually over a number of years and that a history of functional and cognitive decline of only six months is quite likely to be due to another cause. ICD-10 dementia criteria have been modified for use in adults with intellectual disabilities (DC-LD criteria) [16]. As in the general population, ICD-10 criteria are likely to be less inclusive than DSM-IV criteria, primarily because of the additional requirement of a decline in emotional control or behaviour [17].

11.6 Epidemiology

Although some studies have indicated that older adults with intellectual disabilities have rates of dementia similar to that of the general population, a few studies have suggested increased prevalence rates, even when adults with Down's syndrome are excluded. Some estimates of dementia prevalence in the intellectual disability population without Down's syndrome have been as high as 20% in those aged 65 or older, which is two to three times higher than in the equivalent general older population [18]. However, several methodological issues including representativeness of samples, ascertainment methods, diagnostic criteria and inclusion or exclusion of different sub-types hamper research in this area.

A number of factors could increase the risk of dementia in people with intellectual disabilities including reduced brain reserve, which may bring forward the stage at which a person with brain pathology presents with symptoms, lack of educational and cognitively stimulating activity, physical exercise and comorbidities such as epilepsy and head injury. Factors that may reduce the risk for dementia in people with intellectual disabilities include increased mortality in those with more severe disability or comorbidity, giving rise to a healthy cohort effect and lower rates of smoking and substance abuse.

A number of genetic syndromes are associated with hypertension, diabetes, hyperhomocysteinuria and hyperlipidaemia potentially increasing the risk of vascular dementia. Rare syndromes such as Sanfilippo syndrome (mucopolysaccharoidosis III) and Cockayne syndrome (progeria-like-syndrome), a rare autosomal recessive disorder, are characterized by premature ageing, including dementia in adulthood [14].

People with Down's syndrome are at high risk of early onset Alzheimer's disease. By the age of 40 years most adults with Down's syndrome have neuropathology consistent with Alzheimer's disease. Triplication of the amyloid precursor protein gene on chromosome 21 results in increased levels of amyloid precursor protein and deposition of amyloid β fragments as the person ages. Other genes on chromosome 21 may also contribute to the risk of Alzheimer's disease. However, not everyone with Down's syndrome develops dementia. The average age at diagnosis is between 50 and 55 years, several decades earlier than the onset of Alzheimer's disease in the general population. Those in their fifth decade have a 9% rate of dementia, which increases exponentially with ageing so that 30–40% of those aged 50–59 are diagnosed [10, 19]. There may be a slight decline in prevalence in the seventh decade which is probably due to the increased mortality associated with dementia, as the incidence of dementia continues to increase steeply [10]. The incidence of dementia may be as high as 25% over 18 months in those aged 40 and older [20].

11.7 Screening for dementia in older people with intellectual disabilities

There are two types of tests that can be used to screen for suspected dementia in people with intellectual disabilities. However, tests based on the performance of individuals, for example the mini-mental state examination (MMSE) are used to screen for dementia in the general population, but are difficult to apply in the intellectual disability population due to varying ability – and those with less ability may not be able to complete tests (floor effects). Nevertheless several tests have been adapted for use in the intellectual disability population [21]. Threshold scores for single applications have not been established and, at present, these tools are best used in sequential assessment rather than screening.

An alternative is to use tools completed by or with caregivers to screen for possible dementia cases. Examples of such tests include the dementia screening questionnaire for individuals with intellectual disabilities (DSQIID) [22] and adaptive behaviour dementia questionnaire (ABDQ) [23]. These tests may be limited by reliability of informants, recall bias and how long the informant has known the person, and it is important to note that screening is not a substitute for a comprehensive clinical assessment.

11.8 Presentation and diagnosis of dementia in people with intellectual disabilities

In general the presentation of dementia in people with mild to moderate intellectual disability is similar to the general population. For example Alzheimer's disease presents with decline in memory and gradually progresses to involve other cortical cognitive functions resulting in decline in activities of daily living. Dementia in adults with more severe intellectual disabilities may be difficult to diagnose due to the severity of lifelong cognitive deficits and may present later with marked functional decline and neurological symptoms such as incontinence, epilepsy and loss of mobility.

The presentation of Alzheimer's disease in people with Down's syndrome has much in common with the presentation of Alzheimer's disease in the general population including rapid forgetting of new learning, word finding difficulties and other language impairments, dyspraxia and loss of visual spatial skills. However, there are important differences. The early presentation of Alzheimer's disease in people with Down's syndrome is characterized by behavioural and personality changes in combination with decline in executive functioning [24]. These 'frontal lobe'-related features are usually manifest later in the course of dementia among the general population. The problem in making an early diagnosis of Alzheimer's disease in Down's syndrome is that personality and behavioural change such as loss of motivation and slowness are non-specific and general functional decline in an older adult with Down's syndrome must not be assumed to be due to Alzheimer's disease.

Up to half of individuals with Down's syndrome and dementia may present with neurological symptoms, such as seizures (generalized and myoclonic) and incontinence, which are normally signs of advanced disease in the general population, suggesting that dementia presents atypically in Down's syndrome, or reflecting the difficulties in making an early diagnosis. Epilepsy and myoclonus become increasingly more common and severe as the disease progresses.

The principles of assessment and diagnosis of dementia in the general population apply. However, the challenge in the assessment of people with intellectual disabilities lies in obtaining a valid longitudinal history from informants, demonstrating a baseline of prior functioning, demonstrating decline in specific cognitive domains and teasing out the contribution to cognitive and functional decline of comorbid conditions. The perception of decline and the way it manifests will depend on the previous level of functioning and pattern of cognitive abilities, and the environmental demands placed on the person.

An essential first step in dementia assessment is to obtain a history from one or more informants who have known the person for some time. The history should be detailed and focused on the onset, nature and temporal progression of functional decline, memory and other cognitive functions, personality and behavioural changes as well as the relevant medical and family history. Every effort should be made to establish a prior baseline of functioning by careful informant interview supplemented with information from medical and other records such as IQ and other psychological tests of cognition, previous functional assessments, or even examples of writing, art and craft work.

The interview with the informant should establish if there has been a decline in baseline in the person's abilities. The CAMDEX-DS [25, 26] contains a structured interview and includes questions to elicit symptoms in many cognitive domains relevant to dementia diagnosis in the individual.

The domains of functioning that should be questioned in detail are shown in Box 11.1 [27].

Additional memory tests may need to be used, such as object memory tasks [28]. The lack of norms means that serial cognitive assessments over time may be required

Box 11.1   Cognitive assessment

1. Executive skills

   a. organizing, sequencing and completing complex tasks (such as getting dressed or making a cup of tea)

2. Memory

   a. remembering the answer to questions asked – for example they may repeatedly ask the same question, though this needs to be distinguished from anxiety

   b. remembering what they did this morning or yesterday

   c. remembering that they have already done something – for example they may do it again

   d. remembering where they have put things

   e. remembering names of people

3. Language skills

   a. finding familiar words

   b. using complex sentences

   c. understanding what has been said

   d. participating in conversations

   e. literacy skills

4. Recognition of objects and people

5. Visual-spatial and constructional skills

   a. finding their way along streets that previously were well known

   b. finding their own room or the toilet

c. negotiating patterned floors or moving from one floor surface to another

d. negotiating stairs, curbs, escalators

e. complexity and detail in drawing, artwork or crafts such as knitting

6. Learnt motor skills

a. dressing and doing up shoe laces, zips and buttons

b. folding and hanging up clothes

c. using cutlery

7. Psychological and behavioural symptoms of dementia

a. loss of motivation

b. sleep disturbance

c. wandering

d. agitation

e. resistiveness

f. irritability and aggression

g. mood changes – for example depression or lability of emotions

h. delusions and hallucinations.

to establish progression of cognitive impairments. Comprehensive neuropsychological and neurological assessment of suspected dementia cases contributes to diagnosis and sub-typing, describing cognitive deficits in order to plan care and can track progression and response to interventions. The CAMDEX-DS [25, 26] contains a comprehensive neuropsychological assessment. However, it does have significant floor effects in some items, and does not establish the presence of rapid forgetting of newly learnt material, a key feature of Alzheimer's disease.

Serial neuroimaging of the brain can identify progressive brain change due to a neurodegenerative disorder, but a single scan may be difficult to interpret due to developmental brain abnormalities. Abnormal EEG findings are generally non-specific and therefore not particularly useful as a dementia diagnostic tool. Nevertheless, these investigations are often required to exclude other causes of cognitive or functional decline, or to demonstrate cerebrovascular disease.

Comorbid conditions are common in older adults with intellectual disabilities and may be the cause of observed cognitive decline or complicate the presentation – people with multiple health problems are more likely to develop dementia. Careful physical examination and medical workup is essential to identify or rule out comorbid medical conditions (Box 11.2). The identification of vascular risk factors indicates risk for cerebrovascular disease and vascular dementia. Vision and hearing should be checked. Medications should be reviewed, especially sedating medications and anticholinergic medications (often prescribed for extrapyramidal side effects or for urinary incontinence). Serum levels of anticonvulsants should be checked.

Box 11.2   Differential diagnosis of functional decline

- Delirium

- Medication effects, for example antipsychotics, anticholinergics, anticonvulsants

- Other neurological disorders, for example stroke or Parkinson's disease

- Endocrine disorders, for example hypothyroidism, especially in adults with Down's syndrome

- General decline due to other health problems, for example cancer or cardio-vascular disorders or arthritis

- Mental health problems, for example depression

- Sensory impairments.

Mental illness such as depression may cause significant cognitive and functional decline (pseudodementia). Onset of functional decline over months rather years is more likely to be depression than dementia. However, depression may be a symptom of dementia. A history of depression is more common in people with Down's syndrome with dementia than in those without dementia [10, 29].

Case vignette 11.3

Ellen has Down's syndrome and shares a house with several other people with intellectual disabilities. She has well developed social skills and enjoys the company of other people. She is an accomplished artist, who had participated in several exhibitions of her colourful paintings. At the age of 44, Ellen became confused when she had a urinary tract infection and associated urinary incontinence for which she was prescribed an anticholinergic medication. Her carers noticed memory problems and decline in functioning (she required more assistance in the bathroom and toilet) once the infection cleared. Ellen was referred to a memory clinic. She was assessed with the Dementia scale for Adults with Mental Retardation (DMR) (a carer rated dementia symptom scale) and the CAMDEX-DS. Ellen had some memory impairment on testing, but her overall cognitive functioning was judged to be in keeping with her level of ability on history or testing. Anticholinergic medication for incontinence was stopped and reassessment after six months demonstrated improvement in memory and function.

It is important to identify and manage these other causes of functional decline in conjunction with serial cognitive and functional assessments. For example a treatment trial with an antidepressant medication may result in significant functional and cognitive improvement.

11.9 Management

Dementia is an important diagnosis and care must be taken not to misdiagnose it as decisions about care and services may be made on the basis of the diagnosis. If uncertain a diagnosis of dementia may need to be deferred. Nevertheless, early diagnosis is important for future planning and for treatment. When disease modifying treatments for Alzheimer's disease eventually become available, early diagnosis will assume a higher level of importance.

Pharmacological treatment of dementia

Treatment with the cholinesterase inhibitors – donepezil, rivastigmine and galantamine – or the NMDA receptor antagonist memantine should be considered for Alzheimer's disease. The cholinesterase inhibitors are also useful in Lewy body dementia [30]. None of these medications has been demonstrated to be disease modifying. There is currently limited evidence available for the efficacy of these medications in people with intellectual disabilities [14]. The principles for using these medications in older adults with intellectual disabilities are similar to that in the general population including monitoring of response and side effects. Cholinesterase inhibitors are not so well tolerated in people with Down's syndrome and often need to be discontinued because of side effects including ongoing gastrointestinal symptoms and listlessness. All of these medications may precipitate seizures. Dosage regimes should be adjusted to take account of the small build of people with Down's syndrome.

Pharmacological management of behavioural and psychological symptoms of dementia is beyond the scope of this chapter. The general principles are the same as for the general population, although people with intellectual disabilities may be more prone to adverse effects, require smaller doses and need careful monitoring. Antidepressant medications should be considered if depressive symptoms are present. Antipsychotics, to treat behavioural problems, should be used only as last resort. Myoclonic jerking and seizures need to be treated with anti-epileptic drugs (see Case vignette 11.5). It is also important to recognize and treat infections such as respiratory and urinary tract infections at an early stage. Psychiatric medications are also discussed in Chapter 14.

Case vignette 11.4

Two years later, Ellen re-presented with a six-month history of memory decline, loss of daily living skills, general slowing and emotional volatility. Carer ratings with the DMR and cognitive performance tests (based on CAMDEX-DS) demonstrated decline on previous testing. She was diagnosed with dementia and, after medical workup, she was offered treatment with a cholinesterase inhibitor. This was started at a low dose, and increased slowly. Medication response was monitored with DMR ratings, and the Test for Severe Impairment, which is less demanding than the CAMDEX-DS. Staff were offered a series of dementia training sessions.

Ellen remained relatively stable on treatment for two years. During this time a co-resident also developed dementia and tended to wander into other people's rooms creating tension in the house. The residents were offered a group education session on dementia (adapted to their needs) to help them understand the changes their friends were experiencing. They became less angry and more likely to assist their friends or to seek staff help.

Non-pharmacological management of dementia

Non-pharmacological interventions can improve a person's quality of life, by relieving distress and confusion, support functioning and maintain social engagement. Day programmes should be reviewed and modified. Occupational therapy assessments can identify equipment and home modifications that will support functioning. Attention to footwear and foot care, mobility supports, one-to-one support when walking or using a wheelchair in the later stages can help to prevent falls. Addressing sensory deficits can also improve functioning, however, it may be difficult to get the person to wear glasses or hearing aids or they may lose them.

Ensuring appropriate support and psychoeducation of families and carers is essential in dementia care to help prevent premature transitions in care [14]. Carers can employ a range of strategies to assist with day-to-day functioning (see Box 11.3). The impact on other residents in a group home also needs to be considered by seeking additional care resources. Education of other residents will help them to understand the changes.

Box 11.3   Interventions and strategies to assist day-to-day functioning in dementia

Minimizing confusion
- Consistent staffing

- Maintain routines

- Use strategies such as redirection

- Avoid confrontation

- Limit the number of choices offered

- Reducing clutter

- Avoid noisy, crowded environments

- Deficits in visual processing may mean that changes in floor surfaces may look like changes in level and shiny floors could look like water.

Improving communication
- Use non-verbal means of communication

  - Use objects of reference, for example a towel to indicate they will be having a shower

  - Show the person what to do

  - Use gestures, for example using a hand gesture to ask the person to stand

  - Use touch-based communication, such as touching the person's hand to prompt them to drink

  - Make use of pictures:

    - To represent people (e.g. staff and friends at day placements)

    - To represent planned activities and routines.

    - As labels on the bedroom door, toilet door, cupboards and so on.

- Use strategies to help the person understand what you are saying:

  - Get a person's attention before trying to communicate a message – call them by their name, touch them gently on the arm, or both

  - Make eye contact

  - Use short complete sentences

  - Give one instruction at a time

  - Pause between instructions and bits of information.

Supporting function
- Keep the person active and socially engaged, but:

  - Reduce demands made on the person.

  - Break tasks into simpler steps

— Support the person to do things for themselves by compensating for skills that are deteriorating or lost, by serving finger foods, laying the person's clothing out, avoiding shoes with laces.

Interventions aimed at maintaining cognition or memory function
- Cognitive stimulation through different modalities – for example music therapy, aromatherapy, dancing, favourite TV programmes.

- Reminiscence work, for example life-story books.

- Reality orientation therapy, for example having a predictable day, being continually and repeatedly told or shown reminders, for example what is happening now and what is going to happen next.

11.10 Issues in advanced dementia care

Ageing in place is an option for people in the general population but demarcation issues between mental health, older adult care and disability services may hinder the provision of cross-sector services. Those with end-stage disease become totally dependent on carers to meet their day-to-day needs. They are generally incontinent, may be unable to walk or feed themselves, be unable to speak and have limited means of non-verbal communication. They may have seizures, contractures of joints and become unresponsive to their environment [31]. They have specific care needs, which include consideration for palliative care and tube feeding. Homes may need considerable adaptation to be suitable for older adults with end-stage dementia – including special beds, hoists and wheelchair accessibility. Carers need additional nursing skills. These issues often result in transfer to a nursing home.

Case vignette 11.5

Over time Ellen slowly deteriorated. She no longer engaged in conversations, though she still used single words at times. The quality of her drawings deteriorated. Scores on sequential assessments dropped. She started refusing to go to the day centre, and was offered an individualized care package, with one-to-one carer sessions for walks to the park and visits to her mother, which she continued to enjoy. Her hearing deteriorated, and although she was given hearing aids, she often lost these. She started having frequent falls and was diagnosed with epilepsy and started on anti-epileptic treatment. The cholinesterase inhibitor was withdrawn and her falls improved.

A referral to an occupational therapist resulted in adaptations to her bathroom (such as handrails), installation of a moveable bed and a movement sensitive floor light. She was issued with an epilepsy alarm on her mattress, and her room was fitted with a sensor to alert night staff if she left her room. A barrier was fitted on the stairs. She was given well fitted, non-slip shoes. With these adaptations in place, staff are confident they would be able to meet her needs and would like to care for her to the end, despite further declines in her abilities.

Older adults with intellectual disabilities are a growing population even though early mortality of those with more severe disability is common. The current cohort of older adults with intellectual disabilities may have had a particular social and environmental experience, which, in developed countries, includes large-scale institutionalization.

Psychological stressors therefore include change associated with physical decline, loss of carers and friends or enforced moves. They are at risk of developing age-associated disorders, and physical health problems and disability are common. Mental illnesses occur in similar rates as in the older as in the younger intellectual disability population. It is important to review those with mental illness or taking psychotropic medication thoroughly and regularly, and health comorbidity need to be considered in treatment choice.

Dementias are common in the older population with intellectual disabilities and adults with Down's syndrome have high rates of early onset Alzheimer's disease. There are clinical challenges in dementia assessments of adults with intellectual disabilities and serial assessments may be required to confirm the diagnosis. There is much that can be done to improve quality of life of a person with intellectual disability and dementia from the time of diagnosis to end-stage palliative care.

References

1. Hollins, S., Attard, M.T. von, Fraunhofer, N. *et al.* (1998) Mortality in people with learning disability: risks, causes, and death certification findings in London. *Developmental Medicine and Child Neurology*, **40** (1), 50–56.
2. Haveman, M.J., Heller, T., Lee, L.A. *et al.* (2009) Report on the State of Science on Health Risks and Ageing in People with Intellectual Disabilities: IASSID Special Interest Research Group on Ageing and Intellectual Disabilities/Faculty Rehabilitation Sciences, University of Dortmund. http://www.iassid.org/iassid/content/view/22/37/.

3. Evenhuis, H.M., Theunissen, M., Denkers, I. *et al.* (2001) Prevalence of visual and hearing impairment in a Dutch institutionalized population with intellectual disability. *Journal of Intellectual Disabilities Research*, **45** (Pt 5), 457–464.

4. Evenhuis, H.M. (1997) Medical aspects of ageing in a population with intellectual disability: III. Mobility, internal conditions and cancer. *Journal of Intellectual Disabilities Research*, **41** (Pt 1), 8–18.

5. Wallace, R.A., Webb, P.M. and Schluter, P.J. (2002) Environmental, medical, behavioural and disability factors associated with Helicobacter pylori infection in adults with intellectual disability. *Journal of Intellectual Disabilities Research*, **46** (Pt 1), 51–60.

6. Wagemans, A.M.A. and Cluitmans, J.J.M. (2006) Falls and fractures: a major health risk for adults with intellectual disabilities in residential settings. *Journal of Practice and Policy in Intellectual Disabilities*, **3** (2), 136–138.

7. Celeste, D. and Zaffuto-Sforza, D.O. (2005) Aging with cerebral palsy. *Physical Medicine and Rehabilitation Clinics in North America*, **16**, 235–249.

8. Angelopoulou, N., Souftas, V., Sakadamis, A. and Mandroukas, K. (1999) Bone mineral density in adults with Down's syndrome. *European Radiology*, **9** (4), 648–651.

9. Diamond, L.S., Lynne, D. and Sigman, B. (1981) Orthopedic disorders in patients with Down's syndrome. *Orthopedic Clinics of North America*, **12** (1), 57–71.

10. Coppus, A., Evenhuis, H., Verberne, G.J. *et al.* (2006) Dementia and mortality in persons with Down's syndrome. *Journal of Intellectual Disability Research*, **50** (Pt 10), 768–777.

11. Patti, P.J., Amble, K.B. and Flory, M.J. (2005) Life events in older adults with intellectual disabilities: differences between adults with and without Down syndrome. *Journal of Policy and Practice in Intellectual Disabilities*, **2**, 149–155.

12. Cooper, S.A., Smiley, E., Morrison, J. *et al.* (2007) Mental ill-health in adults with intellectual disabilities: prevalence and associated factors. *British Journal of Psychiatry*, **190**, 27–35.

13. Pary, R.J. (1995) Discontinuation of neuroleptics in community-dwelling individuals with mental retardation and mental illness. *American Journal of Mental Retardation*, **100** (2), 207–212.

14. Strydom, A., Lee, L.A., Jokinen, N. *et al.* (2009) Report on the State of Science on Dementia in People with Intellectual Disabilities: IASSID Special Interest Research Group on Ageing and Intellectual Disabilities, http://www.iassid.org/iassid/content/view/22/37/.

15. World Health Organization (1992) The ICD-10 Classification of Mental and Behavioural Disorders: Clinical Descriptions and Diagnostic Guidelines, World Health Organization, Geneva.

16. Royal College of Psychiatrists (2001) *DC-LD: Diagnostic Criteria for Psychiatric Disorders for Use with Adults with Learning Disabilities/Mental Retardation*, Royal College of Psychiatrists.

17. Strydom, A., Livingston, G., King, M. and Hassiotis, A. (2007) Prevalence of dementia in intellectual disability using different diagnostic criteria. *The British Journal of Psychiatry*, **191**, 150–157.

18. Cooper, S. (1997) High prevalence of dementia among people with learning disabilities not attributable to Down's syndrome. *Psychological Medicine*, **27** (3), 616.

19. Holland, A., Hon, J., Huppert, F.A. *et al.* (1998) Population-based study of the prevalence and presentation of dementia in adults with Down's syndrome. *The British Journal of Psychiatry*, **172** (6), 498.

20. Holland, A.J., Hon, J., Huppert, F.A. and Stevens, F. (2000) Incidence and course of dementia in people with Down's syndrome: findings from a population-based study. *Journal of Intellectual Disability Research*, **44** (Pt 2), 138–146.
21. Pyo, G., Kripakaran, K., Curtis, K. *et al.* (2007) A preliminary study of the validity of memory tests recommended by the Working Group for individuals with moderate to severe intellectual disability. *Journal of Intellectual Disability Research*, **51** (5), 377–386.
22. Deb, S., Hare, M., Prior, L. and Bhaumik, S. (2007) Dementia screening questionnaire for individuals with intellectual disabilities. *British Journal of Psychiatry*, **190**, 440–444.
23. Prasher, V., Farooq, A. and Holder, R. (2004) The Adaptive Behaviour Dementia Questionnaire (ABDQ): screening questionnaire for dementia in Alzheimer's disease in adults with Down syndrome. *Research in Developmental Disabilities*, **25** (4), 385–397.
24. Ball, S.L., Holland, A.J., Treppner, P. *et al.* (2008) Executive dysfunction and its association with personality and behaviour changes in the development of Alzheimer's disease in adults with Down syndrome and mild to moderate learning disabilities. *British Journal of Clinical Psychology*, **47** (Pt 1), 1–29.
25. Ball, S., Holland, A., Huppert, F.A. *et al.* (2006) *CAMDEX-DS: The Cambridge Examination for Mental Disorders of Older People with Down's syndrome and Others with Intellectual Disabilities*, Cambridge University Press, Cambridge.
26. Ball, S.L., Holland, A.J., Huppert, F.A. *et al.* (2004) The modified CAMDEX informant interview is a valid and reliable tool for use in the diagnosis of dementia in adults with Down's syndrome. *Journal of Intellectual Disability Research*, **48** (Pt 6), 611–620.
27. Torr, J., Iacono, T., Rickards, L. and Winters, D. (2009) About Down Syndrome and Alzheimer's Disease, Sydney Alzheimer's Australia.
28. Sano, M., Aisen, P., Dalton, A. *et al.* (2005) Assessment of aging individuals with Down syndrome in clinical trials: results of baseline measures. *Journal of Policy and Practice in Intellectual Disabilities*, **2** (2), 126–138.
29. Burt, D., Primeaux-Hart, S., Loveland, K. *et al.* (2005) Tests and medical conditions associated with dementia diagnosis. *Journal of Policy and Practice in Intellectual Disabilities*, **2** (1), 56.
30. Bhasin, M., Rowan, E., Edwards, K. and McKeith, I. (2007) Cholinesterase inhibitors in dementia with Lewy bodies: a comparative analysis. *International Journal of Geriatric Psychiatry*, **22** (9), 890–895.
31. Cosgrave, M., Tyrrell, J., McCarron, M. *et al.* (2000) A five year follow-up study of dementia in persons with Down's syndrome: early symptoms and patterns of deterioration. *Irish Journal of Psychological Medicine*, **17** (1), 11.

Further reading

National Institute for Clinical Excellence (NICE) (2006) Dementia: Supporting People with Dementia and Their Carers in Health and Social Care, http://www.nice.org.uk/CG42.
Down Syndrome Association http://www.downs-syndrome.org.uk/.

12 Management of Offenders with Intellectual Disabilities

Evan Yacoub and Ian Hall

East London NHS Foundation Trust, UK

12.1 Introduction

Like other people in society, people with intellectual disabilities sometimes commit criminal offences. In this chapter, after reviewing the background literature, we outline how to assess offenders with an intellectual disability including discussion of some specific legal issues that they can face. We then discuss how people with intellectual disabilities can be supported to overcome offending behaviours and how services can be configured to meet such needs.

12.2 Background

What is offending behaviour?

Holland *et al.* have reviewed the issues associated with the defining 'criminal offending' in relation to people with intellectual disabilities [1]. Identifying illegal behaviour or consequence is one aspect, sometime called the *actus rea*. However, the definition of more serious offences (such as murder, rape and arson) often requires the intent to perform the act or bring about its consequences, sometimes called the *mens rea* or guilty mind. In contrast, to convict people of more minor offences such as many motoring offences, it is only necessary to prove the *actus rea*, and not that there was *mens rea* [2].

Intellectual Disability Psychiatry: a practical handbook   Angela Hassiotis, Diana Andrea Barron and Ian Hall (eds)
© 2009 John Wiley & Sons, Ltd

For people with intellectual disabilities, it can be a major issue to decide whether there was intent, and expert evidence can be called to help determine this. Do 'offenders' with intellectual disabilities always know what they were doing, or what the consequences of their actions might be?

Prevalence of offending in people with intellectual disabilities

Hodgins probably performed the best study of the prevalence of offending in people with intellectual disabilities [3]. She looked at convictions for a Swedish birth cohort of over 15 000 people born in Stockholm in the same year who were followed up for 30 years. She concluded that men with an intellectual disability (identified through attending special classes) were three times as likely to be convicted as men without intellectual disability, and women with an intellectual disability were four times more likely to be convicted than women without intellectual disabilities.

The extent to which higher conviction rates in people with intellectual disabilities result from differences in arrest (caused, e.g. by intellectually disabled offenders being less able to evade the police) rather than differences in offending is unclear [4]. Simpson and Hogg comment that the prevalence of offending among people with intellectual disabilities compared with the general population is impossible to assess firmly on the available information, and that further research is required [5].

Baron *et al.* found that intellectually disabled offenders start offending at an early age, that they frequently have a history of multiple offences, and that sex offending and arson are over-represented offence types [6]. The latter finding has been replicated in other studies although Simpson and Hogg reported that it was in clients with borderline intellectual functioning (IQs of 71–84) rather than intellectual disabilities where this over-representation took place.

Coid, in a retrospective study of 362 men remanded to a UK prison for psychiatric reports, found that approximately 10% had a learning disability [7]. Rack notes that '20% of the prison population have some form of hidden disability which will affect and undermine their performance in both education and work settings' [8]. It is anticipated that more will be known about the prevalence of learning disability in UK prisons with the publication of the full results of the *No One Knows* programme implemented by the Prison Reform Trust [9].

Female offenders with intellectual disabilities

A study of the characteristics of a cohort of female patients referred to a forensic intellectual disability service found that: [10]

• Females constitute 9% of referrals to the service.

- The history of sexual abuse (61%) in the cohort of female offenders is higher than in male cohorts but at 38.5% physical abuse is no higher than in appropriate comparison groups.

- Identification of mental illness is high at 67%.

- Total reoffending over five years was 22% but, excluding prostitution, was only 16.5%.

It was concluded that in some respects, this cohort of female offenders shows similar characteristics to their male counterparts. However, there are higher levels of mental illness, higher levels of sexual abuse and lower levels of reoffending. It was hypothesized that as females constitute such a low percentage of referrals, it suggests that women with intellectual disabilities do not show the same levels of sexually abusive behaviour or aggressive behaviour – the two most frequent reasons for male referral. Therefore, an intervening variable such as mental illness may indeed be a significant factor. Lower reoffending rates may indicate the success of interventions directed at psychological problems and mental illness.

Forensic intellectual disability psychiatry

Johnston and Halstead described the practice of forensic psychiatry in the intellec-tually disabled population as having distinct but subtle differences from general forensic and mental health services, and as a blend of the philosophies and styles of two cultures [11]. They point out that the literature base for forensic intellectual disability psychiatry remains sparse, and that low prevalence rates, low research funds for this minority group, ethical research restrictions and the diversity of service provision have militated against large-scale surveys of this offender population. They also raise the dilemma that many behaviours have been regarded as 'challenging' rather than 'forensic', although the severity of the resultant interpersonal or property damage might differ little.

Although the evidence base in this sub-specialty is expanding, it remains relatively small particularly in terms of robust randomized controlled trials.

Secure intellectual disability services

Many offenders with intellectual disabilities have been judged to require institutional care outside the prison system, and have been looked after in secure institutions. In England, for example, Broadmoor and Moss Side special hospitals were built, and took large numbers of people with intellectual disabilities. Some time later 'high secure care' for people with intellectual disabilities was taken over by Rampton hospital, which was built in 1912.

In England, from the mid-1970s it was recognized that in addition to high security hospitals and prisons, there was a need for more local, medium secure care for some offenders with intellectual disabilities [12]. This has gradually been implemented although the development of special secure services for offenders with intellectual disabilities has been uneven [13]. In more recent times, much of the provision has been in the independent sector, that is not directly provided by the state-run health service [14, 15].

One needs assessment of a regionally defined group of intellectually disabled forensic patients found them to be a heterogeneous group with wide-ranging psychiatric needs [16]. The majority were cared for outside their geographical area of origin, either in specialist state-run facilities or the independent sector. Those with an additional diagnosis of mental illness were most likely to be detained in state facilities within the region; a diagnosis of personality disorder was associated with placement in either a high secure setting or the independent sector.

This needs assessment also found that individuals with a clinical diagnosis of intellectual disabilities (who were male, and had no additional diagnosis) were most likely to be detained in services provided by specialist intellectual disabilities/mental health trusts out of area. There was a small group of women who were all placed outside the region. Offending behaviour was most likely to consist of violence against the person, sexual offences and arson. The majority assessed were felt to have long-term needs. The study raised important implications for future provision of forensic services in the area, particularly the need to offer services with treatment programmes tailored to the needs of the population under review.

12.3 Assessment

Assessing offenders with intellectual disabilities

The general principles of assessing people with intellectual disabilities apply (see Chapters 2 and 3). These include:

1. Ensuring good communication, by using clear sentences and testing comprehension. For example, assessing whether people know what the words used to describe their offence mean, such as 'grievous bodily harm'.
2. Using accessible information where possible. The use of diagrams and pictures can be very useful, such as a picture of weapons which are illegal to carry.
3. Repeated assessments, as increased familiarity may lead to a better rapport.
4. The use of familiar settings where possible. For example, seeing people not in custody at a centre they are familiar with, or at home (dependent on risks).

5. The importance of informants, and enabling the presence of informants at interviews if the client wants this. An example is a key worker of the same gender who the client may confide in.

Case vignette 12.1

A client with intellectual disability known to the local community learning disability service (CLDS) was arrested for carrying a weapon. His dysarthria and difficulties in communication made it difficult for the police doctor to assess his fitness to be interviewed by the police. His local CLDS was contacted, and through the use of diagrams of relevant aspects such a weapon and the police it was ascertained that he was indeed fit to be interviewed. He was aware that weapons are dangerous, and that carrying them can lead others to worry that he may harm people.

There are a number of aspects of the psychiatric assessment which are particularly relevant to offenders with intellectual disabilities:

1. **Current social situation:** support and supervision of people with intellectual disabilities often play a crucial role in the management of risk.
2. **Past psychiatric history:** in particular this may include indicators of impulsivity such as hyperkinetic disorders, or predictors of patterns of behaviour such as ASDs.
3. **Forensic history:** including reported behaviours which would have been deemed as 'offending behaviours' had the victims pursued criminal charges.
4. **Psychosexual history:** particularly where there is evidence of poor sexual knowledge or unsuccessful attempts to establish sexual relationships.

Case vignette 12.2

The death of a carer was followed some weeks later by a service user with intellectual disability being arrested for sexually inappropriate behaviour. Increasing the support package for this service user, and supervising him when he was out (with his agreement) led to the cessation of these behaviours, which were not present when his carer was alive.

The above applies to professionals assessing people identified as having intellectual disabilities. The *No One Knows* programme by the Prison Reform Trust found that the identification of people with intellectual disabilities within the criminal justice system and their diversion out of it are issues which need to be addressed [9]. The report makes a number of recommendations for the assessment of people with intellectual disabilities by police officers:

- A system should be introduced across all police forces for screening suspects for vulnerability, to include identification of difficulties associated with communication and comprehension. Training for custody officers on how to undertake the screening must also be put in place.

- All forces should provide training for all officers, and particularly custody officers, on methods of presenting the caution and legal rights with maximum clarity. For example, officers can be taught to present the caution sentence by sentence if there is any doubt about the suspect's comprehension. Officers should also be encouraged to test suspects' understanding of the caution and legal rights routinely.

Often there are specific safeguards for vulnerable people in the criminal justice system. For example, in England and Wales, the 1984 Police and Criminal Evidence Act established a safeguard for suspects with intellectual disabilities, through the provision of an appropriate adult to advise and assist the suspect during police interview.

Specific legal issues

This chapter cannot hope to cover the specific legal issues that might arise in every case, or in the different jurisdictions where this book is read. However, fitness to plead, mental abnormality as a defence, and disposal options are usually of relevance, and discussed below in relation to English law.

Fitness to plead

Fitness to plead (guilty or not guilty) must be assessed on a case by case basis, and is established using Pritchard criteria:

- Understand the charge (What have you been charged with? What does assault/ robbery, etc. mean?).

- Enter a plea (guilty or not guilty, know its meaning and consequence).

- Follow proceedings (What happens after you're charged?). Understand evidence (What does witness mean?). Instruct lawyer (What is the advantage of having a lawyer to represent you?).

- Challenge a juror (What does jury mean?).

Essentially, does the defendant have the capacity to take part in proceedings to an adequate extent for a fair trial? If the defendant is found unfit to plead, a trial of facts would then take place to make a finding of whether the defendant did the act, and if it is found the defendant did the act, then the sentence is at the discretion of the judge.

This assessment is a dynamic one, and its outcome can change over time. Coaching of a person with learning disability, and an improvement in any mental health condition, can mean that a defendant who is unfit to plead can at a later stage become fit to plead, and vice versa.

Mental abnormality as a defence in court

1. **Not guilty by reason of insanity:** where on a balance of probabilities, the defendant must prove that at the time the offence:

   > He was labouring under such a defect of reason, arising from a disease of the mind, that he did not to know the nature and quality of the act he was doing, or, if he did know it that he did not know that what he was doing was wrong.

   This is referred to as the McNaughten Rules. Intellectual disabilities can be associated with a defect of reason, where the defendant, for example may not be aware what the legal age for sexual consent is, therefore not knowing that what 'he was doing was wrong'. It is important to ensure that a good collateral history is established in such cases as the defendant may deny knowing a particular fact if he or she feel that confessing to knowing may lead to a harsher outcome.
2. **Diminished responsibility:** this is where an abnormality of mind (whether arising from a condition of arrested or retarded development of mind or any inherent causes or induced by disease or injury) is said to have substantially impaired a defendant's mental responsibility for his acts. This defence can reduce a murder charge to one of manslaughter.
3. **Automatism:** automatism occurs when there is a total loss of voluntary control, a state near unconsciousness leading to involuntary non-purposeful acts. This is often associated with epilepsy. Other examples include sleepwalking and dissociation.

Disposal

If a defendant with intellectual disability is found guilty of a crime, the judge would then have a range of options available for sentencing depending on a number of factors, such as the seriousness of the crime, and whether the defendant has a mental disorder. These options can be as: [2]

1. The law takes its course, for example a fine, prison.
2. Conditional or absolute discharge, possibly with voluntary psychiatric treatment.

3. Probation order, with or without condition of psychiatric treatment.
4. Detention under the Mental Health Act. This will be discussed further under 'Management of offenders with intellectual disabilities'.

Risk assessment of offenders with intellectual disabilities

Manthorpe *et al.* define risk as the possibility that a given course of action will not achieve its desired outcome but instead some undesired situation will develop [17]. They point out that people with intellectual disabilities are usually presumed to be less able to evaluate risks than 'fully competent' individuals, and that the benefits of risk are often neglected, such as gaining independence after crossing the road. They discuss the 'risk conundrum' where professional and service user perceptions do not tally. Good practice is described as balancing the promotion of ordinary living against practical issues of safety. This is a dilemma which is faced by professionals working with this service user group on a daily basis.

Risks include:

- Harm to others

- Harm to self – accidental and intentional

- Neglect

- Damage to property

- Exploitation.

There are now several risk assessment tools available that have been evaluated in people with intellectual disabilities. In a review, Gray *et al.* argue that unaided clinical judgement is poor at predicting future dangerousness in mentally disordered offenders, citing Monahan's work in this field [18, 19]. They propose that as a result, a range of instruments have been developed to assess risk (with promising results), based on:

- Personality traits (e.g. Psychopathy Checklist-Revised (PCL-R)). PCL-R is a frequently used tool for assessing psychopathy [20].

- Actuarial models (e.g. Violence Risk Appraisal Guide [VRAG]) [21, 22].

- Structured clinical judgement (e.g. History, Clinical, Risk Management-20 [HCR-20]), a very useful tool for the assessment of violence in clinical settings [23].

These risk assessment instruments have been found to be 'all significant predictors of violent and general reconviction' in a sample of people with an intellectual disability [24].

In terms of predictors of sexual violence risk in people with an intellectual disability, Lindsay *et al.* found that: [25]

- Risk Matrix 2000-C (combined risk of sexual and non-sexual offending) discriminated between groups, with participants from high security having higher scores than those in medium security, who had higher scores than those in the community.

- The Static-99 showed a significant area under the curve for the prediction of sexual incidents.

These are both useful and frequently used tools in clinical practice, and both have now been validated in people with intellectual disabilities. The Questionnaire on Attitudes Consistent with Sexual Offenders (QASCOs) is also a useful assessment instrument specifically designed for people with intellectual disabilities [26, 27].

12.4 Management

Many offenders with intellectual disabilities, like their non-disabled counterparts, come from chaotic backgrounds. Services for offenders with intellectual disabilities, particularly inpatient settings, can bring about positive results by providing much needed structure, as well as a setting where basic skills can be learnt and education can be provided. Services should be multidisciplinary, including the full range of professions including nursing, psychology, psychiatry, occupational therapy, speech and language therapy, creative therapies, social work, teachers and advocacy. Inpatient services should aim to be person centred, local to people's families and social networks, and to promote community reintegration [28]. They also should be integrated with mainstream forensic services where possible. Engagement with families and social networks should be a priority, as should supporting people to develop community skills through focussed sessions and a structured and supported leave programme to the local community. The provision of community outreach to support people after discharge is vital, as is working with local housing providers to develop supported living placements.

Mental health legislation forms a crucial part of managing risk and providing a structure for therapeutic intervention. In England and Wales, inpatients with intellectual disabilities may be voluntary, or under a civil section such as section 3 of the 1983 Mental Health Act [29]. For offenders with intellectual disabilities, there are the so-called 'forensic' orders in Part 3 of the Mental Health Act. However, for treatment orders under the Act, if someone is being detained because of their intellectual disability (rather than another mental disorder), then they must meet the behavioural criterion of 'abnormally aggressive or seriously irresponsible behaviour'.

Courts can make people convicted of a criminal offence subject to a hospital order for treatment, or subject to guardianship, by making an order under section 37. These are alternative 'disposals' when otherwise the outcome might have been, for example a prison sentence. Where a hospital order (section 37) is made in respect of an offender by the Crown court, and it appears to the court that it is necessary for the protection of the public from serious harm so to do, the court may further order that the offender shall be subject to special restrictions. This means that the government minister (the Secretary of State for Justice) has to authorize periods of leave, and eventual discharge. This is known as a restriction order (section 41).

Other relevant Part 3 orders that can be applied to intellectually disabled offenders include:

1. Remand to hospital for reports (section 35).
2. Remand for treatment (section 36).
3. Interim hospital order (section 38), which enables a convicted offender to stay in hospital on the grounds of mental disorder, for 12 weeks initially, and a maximum of 12 months, and is made by a magistrate's or Crown court, to help decide the ultimate 'disposal' for the offender.
4. For offenders in prison, but not before the court, there is transfer to hospital of sentenced prisoner (section 47), or unsentenced prisoner (section 48). Both of these orders may be subject to a restriction order under section 49.

Case vignette 12.3

An inmate with intellectual disability, whose diagnosis and potential to engage with psychological treatment was unclear, was transferred to a secure facility under section 38. This enabled clarification in terms of both factors, and enabled the court to decide later to place him on a hospital order.

For many offenders with intellectual disabilities, therapeutic work that specifically addresses the behaviour that led to the contact with the criminal justice system is helpful and appropriate. This can include work around sexual offending, anger management and fire-setting.

Sexual offences

There is currently no randomized controlled trials evidence to guide the use of interventions for intellectually disabled sex offenders [30]. Behavioural work is one of the most commonly used interventions in service users with intellectual disabilities and sexual offending and involves rewards such as increased access to enjoyable activities. In a thorough theoretical analysis Lindsay reviews the motivation and aetiology of sex offenders with an intellectual disability, and develops a two-stage model of treatment for sex offenders [31]. The first stage addresses motivation and strategies for offending, and the second promotes engagement with society.

Much of the recent literature on treatment has focussed on group interventions. For men without intellectual disabilities, group cognitive behaviour therapy (CBT) is recognized as the leading method of treatment [32]. Some sex offender groups are run specifically for men with intellectual disabilities as they may be excluded from mainstream groups that are not sufficiently accessible. Components of CBT treatment include:

- Enhancing self-esteem.

- Challenging and changing cognitive distortions.

- Developing victim empathy.

- Developing social functioning.

- Modifying sexual preferences.

- Ensuring relapse prevention.

Hays *et al.* interviewed a group of 16 men with intellectual disabilities and sexually abusive behaviour to ascertain their views after completing a one-year group cognitive behavioural treatment for sexual offending [33]. Participants found the following to be the most salient components of treatment: sex education; legal and illegal behaviours and their consequences; and discussions about specific sexual assaults. Craig *et al.* describe a treatment group where participants were diverted from criminal proceedings and attended a seven-months treatment programme comprising sex education, cognitive distortions, offending cycle and relapse prevention [34]. They showed a trend for improvements in sex knowledge and honesty of sexual interest and significant improvements in socialization skills. No further incidents of sexual offending were reported during a 12-month follow-up. This is often thought to be the most important outcome measure.

Anger and aggression

Novaco has carried out a lot of cognitive behavioural work on assessing and managing anger in service users with an intellectual disability over the last two decades [35]. Many of the anger treatment studies in the intellectual disabilities field involve interventions based on Novaco's work. Cognitive restructuring appears to be a core component, focusing on amelioration of cognitive skills. Behavioural skills training has also been identified to be beneficial [36].

Taylor *et al.* carried out a controlled trial in order to investigate the effectiveness of anger management [37]. Detained men with intellectual disabilities and histories of offending were allocated to specially modified cognitive behavioural anger treatment ($n = 9$) or to routine care waiting-list control ($n = 10$) conditions. Eighteen sessions of individual treatment were delivered over a period of 12 weeks. Treatment outcome was evaluated by participants' self-report of anger intensity to an inventory of provocations and by staff ratings of the anger attributes of participants' ward behaviour. They found that the men reported that anger intensity was significantly lower following the anger treatment, compared to the routine care waiting-list condition. There were largely no treatment condition effects in staff-rated anger. Limited evidence for the effectiveness of anger treatment was provided by the staff ratings of participant behaviour post-treatment.

More recently, cognitive behavioural interventions have shown promise, but the mechanisms for effective change have yet to be delineated.

Fire-setting

There is a dearth of evidence to guide assessment and treatment in pathological fire-setters, especially those with intellectual disabilities. Lindsay argues that these patients share life histories of abuse, deprivation and repeated failures in service settings [35].

Chaplin summarizes recent literature on the treatment of fire-setters with intellectual disabilities [26]. A longitudinal study from Finland aimed to characterize arson recidivists by observing 90 arson recidivists including 16 with intellectual disabilities, five of whom had comorbid alcohol dependency. The wider conclusions were that 68% had issues with alcohol and those with intellectual disabilities were more likely to be 'pure arsonists', that is offenders whose only offence was arson [38].

A pilot study was carried out with six female fire-setters and their treatment using cognitive behavioural techniques, delivered over 40 sessions with a two-year follow-up of the participants [39]. The study aimed to examine participants' motivations for setting fires, their responses to an intervention designed specifically for this group and to monitor their progress over an extended follow-up period. The main outcome reported was that no fires were noted to have been set from any of the fire-setters group at the point of follow-up. The methodology was limited in that it did not control for other variables such as risk management plans and their effect and association with outcomes.

Community treatments for offenders with intellectual disabilities

As described elsewhere (also see Chapter 9) services for people with intellectual disabilities look to support people in the least restrictive environment possible, and with modern models of community care, such as day opportunities and activities, supported housing and living and person centred planning [28].

Community forensic teams would typically have the following members:

- A team manager, often from a nursing or social work background.

- Community nurses.

- Social workers.

- A consultant psychiatrist and a junior psychiatrist.

- A clinical psychologist.

Potential sources of referral include community teams, and those referred through the criminal justice system (such as the probation service and the courts). Another important source is people being discharged from local secure units, many of whom may still be subject to mental health legislation, for example including patients on supervised community treatment in England and Wales. Patients likely to benefit from the specialist expertise of a community forensic team for people with intellectual disabilities include:

- Those with complex needs, often including challenging behaviour and/or substance misuse.

- A serious and ongoing risk of violence, sexually inappropriate behaviour, or other harm to others.

Craig *et al.* showed that offenders with intellectual disabilities can be engaged psychologically in the community as well as within secure settings [34]. One of the challenges for secure intellectual disabilities services is liaising with community services in order to ensure that discharges are not delayed, and that they are safe. This is much easier to implement if secure services are local [15].

Regarding offence-specific treatment in the community, Lindsay *et al.* compared the responses to treatment of sex offenders with intellectual disabilities receiving different length probationary sentences [40]. The group treatment addressed issues of: denial, minimization and responsibility for the offence; harm done to the victim;

behaviour consistent with offending; and victim awareness and confidentiality. The subjects were assessed on a standard questionnaire designed to assess attitudes consistent with sex offending. There was a significant difference between the groups at the end of the probation period with subjects sentenced to two years' probation showing greater improvement. The authors recommend that a court order for a one-year period of probation with treatment is of little value when dealing with sex offenders with intellectual disabilities.

There is some information on prognosis for people discharged from specialist units. A follow-up study looking at long-term outcomes for people with intellectual disabilities discharged from a medium secure service found that although challenging behaviours resembling the original offence continued, reconviction rates were low at only 11% [41].

12.5 Conclusion

Forensic intellectual disability psychiatry is a relatively new field with a relatively new and limited evidence base. Some of the assessment and treatment approaches used in mainstream forensic psychiatry can be applied to offenders with intellectual disabilities, but often require a degree of modification to ensure good communication and understanding, and a proper development perspective that allows people to mature and develop their skills. The move towards more local inpatient and community-based services is a positive one, and should help to achieve a more person centred approach that will hopefully deliver better outcomes both for society and for offenders with intellectual disabilities.

References

1. Holland, T., Clare, I. and Mukhopadhyay, T. (2002) Prevalence of 'criminal offending' by men and women with intellectual disability and the characteristics of 'offenders': implications for research and service development. *Journal of Intellectual Disabilities Research*, **46** (1), 6–20.
2. Puri, B.K., Laking, P.J. and Treasaden, I.H. (2002) *Textbook of Psychiatry*, 2nd edn, Churchill Livingstone, Edinburgh, pp. 391–425.
3. Hodgins, S. (1992) Mental disorder, intellectual deficiency and crime: evidence from a birth cohort. *Archives of General Psychiatry*, **49**, 476–483.
4. Robertson, G. (1988) Arrest patterns among mentally disordered offenders. *British Journal of Psychiatry*, **153**, 313–316.
5. Simpson, M.K. and Hogg, J. (2001) Patterns of offending among people with intellectual disability: a systematic review. Part I: methodology and prevalence data. *Journal of Intellectual Disability Research*, **45** (5), 384–396.

6. Baron, P., Hassiotis, A. and Banes, J. (2001) Offenders with intellectual disability: a prospective comparative study. *Journal of Intellectual Disability Research*, **48** (1), 69–76.

7. Coid, J.W. (1988) Mentally abnormal prisoners on remand: rejected or accepted by the NHS? *British Medical Journal*, **296**, 1779–1782.

8. Rack, J. (2005) *The Incidence of Hidden Disabilities in the Prison Population*, Dyslexia Institute, Egham, Surrey.

9. Prison Reform Trust (2007) *No One Knows: Offenders with Learning Difficulties and Learning Disabilities – Review of Prevalence and Associated Needs*, Prison Reform Trust, ISBN 0946209847.

10. Lindsay, W.R., Smith, A.H., Quinn, K. *et al.* (2004) Women with intellectual disability who have offended: characteristics and outcome. *Journal of Intellectual Disability Research*, **48** (6), 580–590.

11. Johnston, S. and Halstead, S. (2000) Forensic issues in intellectual disability. *Current Opinion in Psychiatry*, **13**, 475–480.

12. Home Office and Department of Health and Social Services (1975) *Report of the Committee on Mentally Abnormal Offenders (Butler Report) (Cmnd 6244)*, The Stationery Office, London.

13. Chiswick, D. and Cope, R. (1995) Facilities and Treatment, *Seminars in Practical Forensic Psychiatry*, Gaskell, pp. 164–209.

14. Department of Health (2004) Commissioning Services Closer to Home, Department of Health.

15. Yacoub, E., Hall, I. and Bernal, J. (2008) Secure in-patient services for people with learning disability: is the market serving the user well? *Psychological Bulletin*, **32** (6), 205–207.

16. Crossland, S., Burns, M., Leach, C. and Quinn, P. (2005) Needs assessment in forensic learning disability. *Medicine, Science and the Law*, **45** (2), 147–153.

17. Manthorpe, J., Walsh, M., Alaszewski, A. and Harrison, L. (1997) Issues of risk practice and welfare in learning disability services. *Disability and Society*, **12**, 69–82.

18. Gray, N.S., Fitzgerald, S., Taylor, J. *et al.* (2007) Predicting future reconviction in offenders with intellectual disabilities: the predictive efficacy of VRAG, PCL-SV, and the HCR-20. *Psychological Assessment*, **19**, 474–479.

19. Monahan, J. (1981) *Predicting Violent Behavior: An Assessment of Clinical Techniques*, Sage, Beverly Hills.

20. Hare, R.D. (1991) *The Hare Psychopathy Checklist-Revised*, Multi-Health Systems, Toronto.

21. Quinsey, V.L., Harris, G.T., Rice, M.E. and Cormier, C.A. (1998) *Violent Offenders: Appraising and Managing Risk*, 1st edn, American Psychological Association, Washington, DC.

22. Quinsey, V.L., Jones, B., Book, A.S. and Barr, K.N. (2006) The dynamic prediction of antisocial behavior among forensic psychiatric patients. *Journal of Interpersonal Violence*, **21**, 1539–1565.

23. Webster, C.D., Douglas, K., Eaves, D. and Hart, S.D. (1997) *HCR-20: Assessing Risk for Violence*, 2nd edn, Simon Fraser University, Vancouver.

24. Gray, N., Snowden, R.J., MacCulloch, S. *et al.* (2004) Relative efficacy of criminological, clinical, and personality measures of future risk of offending in mentally disordered offenders: a comparative study of HCR-20, PCL: SV, and OGRS. *Journal of Consulting and Clinical Psychology*, **72** (3), 523–530.

25. Lindsay, W.R., Hogue, T., Taylor, J.L. *et al.* (2008) Risk assessment in offenders with intellectual disability: a comparison across three levels of security. *International Journal of Offender Therapy and Comparative Criminology*, **52** (1), 90–111.

26. Chaplin, E.H. (2006) Forensic aspects in people with intellectual disabilities. *Current Opinion in Psychiatry*, **19** (5), 486–491.

27. Broxholme, S.L. and Lindsay, W.R. (2003) Development and preliminary evaluation of a questionnaire on cognitions related to sex offending for use with individuals who have mild intellectual disabilities. *Journal of Intellectual Disabilities Research*, **47** (6), 472–482.

28. Department of Health (2001) *Valuing People: A New Strategy for Learning Disability for the 21st Century*, The Stationery Office.

29. Department of Health (2008) *Reference Guide to the Mental Health Act 1983*, The Stationery Office.

30. Ashman, L. and Duggan, L. (2008) Interventions for learning disabled sex offenders. *Cochrane Database of Systematic Reviews* 4.

31. Lindsay, W. (2005) Models underpinning treatment for sex offenders with mild intellectual disability: current theories of sex offending. *Mental Retardation*, **43**, 428–441.

32. Hanson, R.K., Gordon, A., Harris, A.J. *et al.* (2002) First report of the collaborative outcome data project on the effectiveness of psychological treatment for sex offenders. *Sexual Abuse: A Journal of Research and Treatment*, **14**, 169–194.

33. Hays, S.J., Murphy, G., Langdon, P. *et al.* (2007) Group treatment for men with intellectual disability and sexually abusive behaviour: service user views. *Journal of Intellectual and Developmental Disability*, **32** (2), 106–116.

34. Craig, L.A., Stringer, L. and Moss, L. (2006) Treating sexual offenders with learning disabilities in the community. *International Journal of Offender Therapy and Comparative Criminology*, **50** (4), 369–390.

35. Lindsay, W.R., Taylor, J.L. and Sturmey, P. (2004) *Offenders with Developmental Disabilities*, John Wiley & Sons, Ltd, Chichester.

36. Rose, J., West, C. and Clifford, D. (2000) Group interventions for anger in people with intellectual disabilities. *Research in Developmental Disabilities*, **21**, 171–181.

37. Taylor, J.L., Novaco, R.W., Gillmer, B. and Thorne, I. (2002) Cognitive – behavioural treatment of anger intensity among offenders with intellectual disabilities. *Journal of Applied Research in Intellectual Disabilities*, **15** (2), 151–165.

38. Lindberg, N., Holi, M.M., Tani, P. and Virkkunen, M. (2005) Looking for pyromania: characteristics of a consecutive sample of Finnish male criminals with histories of recidivist fire-setting between 1973 and 1993. *BioMed Central Psychiatry*, **5**, 47.

39. Taylor, J.L., Robertson, A., Thorne, I. *et al.* (2006) Responses of female fire-setters with mild and borderline intellectual disabilities to a group intervention. *Journal of Applied Research in Intellectual Disabilities*, **19**, 179–190.

40. Lindsay, W.R. and Smith, A.H. (1998) Responses to treatment for sex offenders with intellectual disability: a comparison of men with 1- and 2-year probation sentences. *Journal of Intellectual Disability Research*, **42** (5), 346–353.

41. Alexander, R.T., Crouch, K., Halstead, S. and Piachaud, J. (2006) Long-term outcome from a medium secure service for people with intellectual disability. *Journal of Intellectual Disability Research*, **50** (4), 305–315.

13 Mental Health Crises

Deirdre O'Brady

East London NHS Foundation Trust, UK

13.1 Introduction and context

When considering how to support people with intellectual disability in mental health crises, it is imperative to consider their social context and the support that is available to them. This is covered in detail in Chapter 16 and briefly summarized here.

People with intellectual disabilities make up approximately 2% of the population. They are a heterogeneous group, living for the most part in the community in a wide variety of social care settings. The level of support available to individuals is determined by the degree of cognitive, social and adaptive impairment and varies from 24-hour support by professional carers or family, to complete independence in those with milder cognitive impairment. Social policy in the UK has focussed on enabling people with intellectual disabilities to live in the community, with support as necessary, including to access all mainstream health services when required [1]. This includes access to new services developed under the National Service Framework for Mental Health [2]. In emergency situations this may involve community mental health teams, crisis intervention teams or home treatment teams as appropriate.

Specialist expertise in the assessment and management of psychiatric and behavioural disorder is provided by community intellectual disability teams which are usually multidisciplinary in nature and integrated with social services. They provide consultation to mainstream services across the interfaces of primary and secondary care as well as direct intervention where appropriate.

Intellectual Disability Psychiatry: a practical handbook   Angela Hassiotis, Diana Andrea Barron and Ian Hall (eds)
© 2009 John Wiley & Sons, Ltd

13.2 Vulnerability to crises

People with intellectual disabilities have higher rates of physical and psychiatric morbidity than the general population. In addition they may go into crisis situations owing
to environmental or social precipitants which can present as a psychiatric emergency.
The overall prevalence of psychiatric disorder is between 40 and 45% [3, 4]. This
includes disorders of behaviour and emotions which are associated with impairments
of verbal communication in people with moderate or severe intellectual disabilities.
This is also called 'challenging behaviour' or 'problem behaviour' [5] (Box 13.1).
The detailed management of challenging behaviour is discussed in Chapter 9.

Box 13.1 Challenging behaviour [6]

The prevalence of challenging behaviour is between 12 and 17%.

It is a social construct defined as: 'Culturally abnormal behaviours of such
intensity, frequency or duration that the physical safety of the person or others is
likely to be placed in serious jeopardy . . .'[6]

Up to 48% of people who have challenging behaviour are prescribed antipsychotic medication although they may not have mental illness.

More common in moderate/severe intellectual disability, in males, in autism
and in younger people with intellectual disability.

A new episode of behavioural or psychiatric disorder can present on a
background of chronic behavioural disorder.

13.3 Emergency presentations

Emergencies can present:

- In primary care

- In family homes, residential care settings, day services

- To accident and emergency departments

- To mainstream mental health services, for example to community mental health
  teams

- Via the police who may arrest the person and bring him or her to hospital or the
  police station for assessment.

A common reason for requesting an urgent psychiatric assessment is agitated or aggressive behaviours which are putting the individual or other people at risk. This can include:

- Physical aggression towards self or others

- Deliberate self-harm or suicidal behaviour

- Aggression towards objects in the environment

- Fire-setting

- Inappropriate sexual behaviour or sexual offending

- Antisocial behaviour, for example shoplifting.

    Others presentations may include:

- Self neglect

- Vagrancy/wandering.

13.4 Aetiology

The aetiology of these rather non-specific behavioural presentations is often complex and multifactorial. Because people with intellectual disabilities vary widely with regards to their verbal communication, expression of underlying pain, anxiety or any distress may present as agitated or other behaviours (see Chapters 2 and 3 for further discussion of this).

Diagnostic overshadowing

The presence of intellectual disability, especially in an individual with a history of behavioural disorder, may result in the phenomenon of diagnostic overshadowing, whereby a physical or mental illness presenting as agitation or aggression may go unrecognized if the behaviour is attributed to the presence of intellectual disability alone.

Case vignette 13.1

A general practitioner requests support from a psychiatrist from the intellectual disability team in assessing a 60-year-old woman who has recently moved into a

---

residential care home and registered with his practice. For 36 hours she has been agitated, refusing food, sleeping very little, is incontinent of urine and spending large amounts of time in the bathroom. Attempts by her carers to identify the cause of her behaviour have been prevented by physical aggression taking the form of her throwing objects or lashing out at them. The GP adds that she has Down's syndrome and that in the past she was prescribed antipsychotic medication to manage behavioural disorder but that this was discontinued by her psychiatrist two years previously. Her carers say that they are concerned that she has been talking to herself; they are aware of her psychiatric history and wonder if she has an acute mental disorder.

In this situation there are many potential aetiologies. However, when seen the woman was lying on her bed, holding her lower abdomen. After some persuasion she allowed a brief physical examination which revealed abdominal tenderness. She was supported to attend the local general hospital where a diagnosis of a urinary tract infection was made; following treatment she was discharged to her home. Her carers reported that she requested food and that there was no further disturbance of behaviour.

Case vignette 13.1 illustrates the need to take a systematic approach to the assessment of behavioural or other disturbance in people with intellectual disabilities and it may be helpful to consider problems which may be contributing to the emergency presentation using a *biopsychosocial* model [7].

Biological

Physical illness

- People with intellectual disabilities have more physical illness [8] than the general population which may be under-diagnosed due to poor uptake of primary care.

- Common morbidities occur at greater frequency.

- Conditions may present late or mimic psychiatric disorder, for example reflux oesophagitis and weight loss could be misdiagnosed as depression.

- Pain, injury, infection or any medical or surgical emergency can present with acute behavioural disturbance.

- Dental care may be poor, dental pain or infection may present as, for example self-injury.

Epilepsy

- Has an overall prevalence of 22%, [8] rising to 40% in more severe intellectual disabilities.

- Is associated with increased behavioural and psychiatric disorder.

- Can mimic psychiatric disorder, especially complex partial seizures.

- Anti-epileptic medication may cause behavioural disturbance.

- Anti-epileptic medication may cause cognitive impairment and confusion.

Behavioural phenotypes

Certain syndromes are associated with increased risks of physical and mental disorder which may present as emergencies, for example:

- **Down's syndrome:** hypothyroidism, depression, dementia

- **Fragile X syndrome:** ADHD, depression, self-injury, for example wrist biting

- **Prader-Willi syndrome:** behavioural disorder, anxiety, OCD, psychotic episodes, self-injury especially picking skin.

Medication

Up to 40% of people with intellectual disabilities are prescribed psychoactive medication, which may complicate emergency presentations:

- Medication may mask physical illness.

- It may mask psychiatric illness especially in people with autism or more severe intellectual disabilities.

- It may cause cognitive deterioration or confusional states.

- It may cause behavioural deterioration, for example due to akathasia or other extrapyramidal side effects.

- Changes in medication may contribute to sudden changes in behaviour especially if there is polypharmacy, particularly with anti-epileptic medication.

Psychological

The long-term effects of low self-esteem, dependency and powerlessness may impair the psychological resilience of a person with intellectual disability so that an individual is overwhelmed by:

- Bereavement or loss, for example of family members, carers or significant others in the social network.

- Bullying, and physical and sexual abuse.

- Limited ability to cope with social demands and tasks, for example in work placements or in living independently.

- High expressed emotion in family or carers.

Comorbid mental disorders can also increase this psychological vulnerability. This is particularly so in autism (Box 13.2) which is discussed in detail in Chapter 7.

Box 13.2   Emergency presentations in autism

In emergencies, background behaviours in people with autism may increase in severity, including:

- stereotypies

- over activity

- attention deficits

- ritualistic and compulsive behaviours.

People with autism may develop mental illness:

- They may be at higher risk of affective disorders

- Schizophrenia may occur

- Catatonia has been reported.

Epilepsy is a common comorbidity especially in those with lower intellectual functioning, and may present as a sudden behavioural change.

Higher functioning individuals including those with Asperger's syndrome may present with bizarre behaviours, or sexual offences such as stalking.

Social and environmental

People with intellectual disabilities may have inadequate social support, due to non-recognition or underestimation of need. They may be supported by inexperienced or poorly trained carers who themselves are inadequately supported. Change, relocation or transition of the person with intellectual disabilities can be a substantial cause of distress, especially if poorly planned. Finally, longstanding economic deprivation and unemployment may precipitate a crisis, for example through debt or threat of eviction.

Case vignette 13.2

A 48-year-old man with moderately severe intellectual disability is placed in respite care following his mother's admission to hospital with a hip fracture. For over a week he is agitated and restless, refusing food and frequently going to the front door wanting to leave. He is self-injuring by slapping his head, occasionally running around the building asking for his mother. He responds to reassurance but if left unattended becomes distressed again. He has a history of behavioural disturbance during his adolescence but since then has not required specialist input. His mother (who is widowed) declined day services and his general practitioner says he has only attended for minor ailments over the years.

When seen he is anxious with tearfulness and it is difficult to do a full mental state examination. A working diagnosis of adjustment disorder is made and as required lorazepam is prescribed to be reviewed on a daily basis. He is provided with a one-to-one worker while possessions and photographs are collected from his home. The worker spends time explaining that his mother is in hospital using pictures and photographs which he appears to understand. An intellectual disability nurse visits him daily and after a few days he is supported to visit his mother in hospital. His distress diminishes as he adjusts to the situation. A full assessment of both his and his mother's needs is carried out before they return to their home and she acknowledges the need to plan for his future.

In this case the most relevant interventions following the psychiatric diagnosis were psychosocial. In the short term, by enhancing this man's understanding

> of what had happened, his support team were able to alleviate his distress with
> specialist input provided by the intellectual disability nurse. By assessment of
> both his and his mother's needs, future crises can be planned for. In addition, by
> broadening his social opportunities his dependency on his mother for emotional
> and practical support may be reduced.

13.5 Psychiatric presentations

Because of impairments in verbal communication, people with intellectual disabilities may present in atypical ways and aggression is a common presenting
problem, especially in accident and emergency departments [9]. Once physical
illness is excluded, it is important to assess for psychiatric disorder, as any type
of psychiatric disorder may be occurring. A crucial part of an emergency psychiatric assessment is to try and establish a change from baseline behaviour and
functioning.

Anxiety

Anxiety is a common cause of agitated or aggressive behaviour. The prevalence of
anxiety and depression is higher in people with mild intellectual disabilities than in
the general population and it tends to be chronic [10]. Anxiety may be due to a wide
variety of psychiatric problems including persecutory delusions, auditory or other
hallucinations, disorders of mood, adjustment disorders or PTSD. It may be also
be very prominent in autism with increase in stereotypies and repetitive behaviours
precipitated by, for example disruption of routine including loss.

Overactivity

Overactivity and restlessness may be due to:

- ADHD, autism, delirium, dementia or other organic conditions.

- Mania.

- Medication, for example akathasia or other extrapyramidal side effects may
  cause overactivity if antipsychotics have been given to try and calm the
  situation.

Antisocial and disruptive behaviours

Higher rates of offending behaviour occur in people with mild intellectual disabilities, and offenders with intellectual disabilities have higher rates of psychiatric disorder.

Acts of self-harm

Self-injurious behaviour tends to occur in people with moderate to severe intellectual disabilities and people with autism. It may be due to boredom and an inadequate environment as well as depression. Self-cutting and taking overdoses are more likely in people with mild intellectual disabilities, and can be due to any psychiatric disorder or psychosocial crisis. Rarely, attempts at suicide may also occur. Research into suicidal ideation in people with intellectual disabilities shows that one in three individuals with intellectual disabilities had experienced suicidal ideation in the past – this is comparable to that reported in the general population. Moreover up to 11% of individuals with intellectual disabilities disclosed a previous attempted suicide. Accuracy of data regarding the frequency of completed suicide is variable and ranges from none reported to 17 per 100 000 [11]. Clearly suicidality in this population is an important indicator of mental health needs and should considered within the psychiatric assessment of people with mental illness and intellectual disabilities.

Case vignette 13.3

A 30-year-old man with mild intellectual disability and cerebral palsy is brought to the accident and emergency department by ambulance. In the past two days he has twice attempted self-strangulation by wrapping a television cable around his neck. He lives with his family and is provided with 36 hours of social care per week to access community and social activities. However, this has been reduced to 16 hours per week due to funding constraints and he is distraught. He has a history of depression and anxiety for which he is prescribed medication. He has significant dysarthria which combined with tearfulness and agitation make it difficult to communicate with him.

He is referred to the home treatment team who decide that the risk merits an inpatient episode to which he agrees. On the inpatient unit he is subdued and withdrawn.

The community team for people with intellectual disabilities are consulted. He is known to the speech and language therapist who is able to visit the inpatient unit, giving him reassurance and advising the team on his communication style and abilities. He is fearful that he will become housebound and lose his place on his training course as a result in the cut in hours as owing to a combination

---

of intellectual and physical disability he cannot go out without support. During the course of the admission, information about significant intrafamilial discord emerges. His care manager arranges for his care package to be reinstated for a six-month period; he is discharged with arrangements made for psychology to work with his family along with psychiatric follow-up.

In this situation, mainstream adult mental health services, having responded in the usual way, felt uncertain about communication with this man. His severe dysarthria led them to overestimate his level of cognitive impairment. This was frustrating for him and could have reduced the quality of his care. His speech and language therapist was able to explain that his intellectual disability was in the mild range and ensure that his concerns were adequately addressed. This also included highlighting psychological dysfunction within his family, something that he might have found difficult to explain without the support of someone who understood his communication needs. Following resolution of the crisis phase, psychological and social issues could be addressed by the community intellectual disability team working with his community psychiatrist to reduce future risk.

Emergency psychiatric assessment

Psychiatric assessment is covered in detail in Chapter 3. In crisis situations, the following issues are of particular relevance.

Diagnostic issues

- The current problems may represent the new onset of a disorder, especially of adjustment, mood, anxiety or PTSDs.

- They may be an exacerbation or relapse of pre-existing conditions.

- They may be occurring on a background of chronic behavioural disorder.

Information gathering

Wherever assessment occurs, in a crisis it is especially important to get as much background information as possible [12].

- If not already involved, contact the general practitioner.

- Family members or carers are an invaluable source of knowledge, but bear in mind that they may be the source of or contributing to the presentation.

- If in the accident and emergency department, check the records. The person may be well known: some people with intellectual disability are regular attenders, usually because of inadequate social support [9].

- Contact the local community intellectual disability team; even if they don't know the person they may be able to give advice or join you in the assessment.

Immediate risk management and de-escalation

In crisis situations there is often a sense of panic which can be counterproductive to finding the optimal way forward. It is important to:

- Be calm and reassuring, and take time to explain your role.

- Assess or enquire about the level of communication the person with intellectual disability had prior to presentation.

- Use a quiet room free from interruption and distractions.

- Ensure the room is safe, for example free of moveable objects which are potential missiles.

- A trusted carer can help reduce anxiety and agitation.

- Establishing any kind of rapport may take time and patience.

- If the situation allows, see the person alone for part of the assessment. This may reveal situations such as abuse.

If the situation remains volatile, psychotropic medications can be considered. As discussed in Chapter 14, they should be used cautiously as side effects and paradoxical reactions can occur. With this proviso light sedation (such as lorazepam 1 mg) can be given if consent is given, and haloperidol, risperidone or olanzapine may also be helpful. Interventions such as physical restraint or forcible administration of tranquillizing medications are not recommended in most community settings.

Extreme risk

- May require support from the emergency services, that is police or ambulance.

- May require use of the mental health legislation for assessment and/or treatment if the person needs management in psychiatric hospital and does not consent to it. There may be restrictions on using mental health legislation on grounds of their learning disability alone (see Box 13.3).

Box 13.3 Treating someone with a 'learning disability' (intellectual disability) under Mental Health Act in England and Wales

Mental Health Act 1983 (England and Wales, as amended in 2007).
    Mental disorder means 'any disorder or disability of mind'.
    BUT, for treatment orders:

A person with a learning disability 'shall not be considered *by that disability* to be suffering from mental disorder'

UNLESS

that 'disability is associated with abnormally aggressive or seriously irresponsible conduct on his part'.

However, people with learning disability can be detained in any case for treatment of other mental disorders such as mental illness.
    The 'medical treatment' must be for the purpose of alleviating, or preventing a worsening of a mental disorder. This specifically includes nursing and psychological intervention.

Mental state examination

In extreme crises the mental state examination may be limited, but it is important to do as much as possible in crisis situations as the findings can substantially influence outcome. The following aspects are of particular relevance.

Appearance and behaviour

Note dysmorphic features, since a phenotype could point towards behaviour disorder. Neglect may be due to poor adaptive skills or secondary to abuse.

Evidence of alcohol use may be present. Irritability may be due to mania or organic conditions.

Speech

Note verbal ability, level of comprehension and usual style of communication. Dysarthria, echolalia and perseveration may all be present.

Mood

Subjective accounts of mood may be difficult to obtain. Low mood can cause irritability or agitation. Some people have alexithymia, others may complain of physical symptoms. Carers may be able to give information about recent changes in sleep, weight or appetite. Statements of intent to self-harm and or suicidal ideation or intent need to be explored.

Thought

Complaints of persecution may be psychotic in origin or may be reality-based, for example in cases of physical or other abuse. In people with autism obsessive thoughts and compulsions occur, and these may increase in severity and intensity in a crisis.

Perception

Many people with intellectual disabilities talk to themselves or have magical thinking, depending on level of development. Auditory hallucinations may be ill formed, or may be expressed by self-injury, for example striking of the head.

Cognition

The Mini Mental State Examination is not validated for use in people with intellectual disabilities [13]. In emergencies the issue is to establish change from baseline cognitive functioning and exclude or confirm delirium. Confusion may be due to epilepsy. Enquire about recent changes in medication.

Insight

This may be impaired owing to underlying intellectual disabilities as well as mental illness. A person's capacity to consent to interventions must be considered in emergency situations. The law in general is discussed in Chapter 4, and its specific application in crisis management in Box 13.4.

Box 13.4   Capacity in crisis management

Capacity (The Mental Capacity Act 2005, England and Wales)
    The presumption of capacity applies to those with intellectual disabilities, but in emergencies:

- Capacity may be difficult to assess or demonstrate.

- Capacity may be temporarily absent, for example in psychosis or extreme anxiety.

- There may not be time to maximize decision making capacity.

- Interventions must be according to person's best interests.

- Least restrictive options may not be available in an emergency.

    Passive accepting of admission to a psychiatric unit is not the same as giving informed consent and in England and Wales the Mental Health Act (1983) should be applied if consent is lacking.

Diagnosis

Where verbal communication is good (e.g. in many people with mild intellectual disabilities) a psychotic or other disorder may be obvious. However, a definitive diagnosis may not be possible in an emergency when:

- Physical illness cannot be excluded.

- Level of intellectual disability is moderate or severe.

- Autism is present.

- There is a pre-existing history of behaviour disorder.

- Further multidisciplinary assessment is required, for example with a speech and language therapist or a psychologist.

    Containing risk may be the primary concern pending diagnostic clarification and depends on:

- The nature and severity of disorder and associated risk

- The level of underlying intellectual disabilities and adaptive skills

- The degree of social support

- Whether to use adult mental health or specialist intellectual disability services where available, or a combination of both.

Case vignette 13.4

A 19-year-old man is brought to the accident and emergency department by police having been arrested for breaking the windows of his neighbour's flat and shouting at them from the street. He has lived alone for six months with weekly visits from a support worker. He is self-neglected with evidence of weight loss. The police say that his flat is squalid, with no food in the fridge and the electricity has been cut off. The young man complains that his neighbours have been talking about him, which he can hear through his radiators, and that they are responsible for his electricity being cut off. He is preoccupied, muttering to himself and seems slightly thought disordered. He is known to social services having been raised in care but has not been referred to the specialist intellectual disability team. He agrees to an admission to the adult mental health unit for further evaluation of his mental state, allowing specialist intellectual disability services time to contribute to the assessment and advise in planning his future care.

In Case vignette 13.4 and similar situations, the use of mainstream adult mental health services is appropriate and should be actively considered [14, 15].

This might include options such as:

- Referral to the home treatment team

- Referral to an early intervention in psychosis service

- Informal admission to a mainstream psychiatric unit

- Compulsory admission for assessment using the Mental Health Act.

Input from specialist services may be available, for example a community intellectual disability nurse with expertise in mental health may be available to work with mainstream mental health services. They can help differentiate problems arising due to intellectual disabilities and adaptive impairment from those due to mental illness. They can also attend ward rounds and care programme approach meetings and help in clarifying whether follow-up should include input from specialist services.

Case vignette 13.5

A 36-year-old man is brought to the accident and emergency department by his carers. He has moderately severe intellectual disability, autism and a history of behavioural disorder. He is on risperidone to manage his aggressive behaviours. For the past week he has been extremely disruptive, causing extensive damage to his home, breaking furniture and throwing televisions. His carers say that he is unmanageable. There has been no change in sleep, weight or appetite. In between episodes he is described as his usual self and his carers comment that he appears to be 'enjoying' his outbursts. He passively acquiesces with a brief physical examination and seems to be in good health. He presents as calm, his speech is repetitive and echolalic and he is unable to discuss recent events. It is not possible to assess his insight. Admission to psychiatric hospital is being considered. The advice given by the specialist intellectual disability team is that in the absence of obvious mental illness he should return home, with extra levels of support, to be followed up within 24 hours by psychology and psychiatry from the intellectual disability team. It subsequently emerges that following a change in management at his placement, guidelines and protocols for managing his aggressive behaviours are not being followed.

In Case vignette 13.5 and similar situations the role of mainstream mental health services may be limited to initial assessment and exclusion of mental illness. Adult mental health inpatient units may not be resourced to manage people with moderate or severe intellectual disabilities and admission could even put them at risk. Furthermore many intellectual disability teams include a community mental health team or an assertive outreach team [15] who can work with people who have complex comorbidities such as autism.

Specialist inpatient units for people with intellectual disabilities may be available but admission may not be available immediately. Occasionally someone has to be admitted to a mainstream unit and transferred as soon as practicable. However, it is usually helpful to consider a range of other options first: respite care may be available, or increased support can be provided to where the person lives allowing time for multidisciplinary assessment of the problem.

13.6 Summary

Psychiatric crises in intellectual disabilities present in a variety of ways, often non-specifically. Aetiology may be complex and multifactorial. Management should utilize mainstream services where appropriate, with the support of specialist intellectual disability services. They provide advice and consultation to mainstream services, with direct intervention as appropriate, especially for more challenging and complex cases. Figure 13.1 gives a simplified version of the approach described in this chapter.

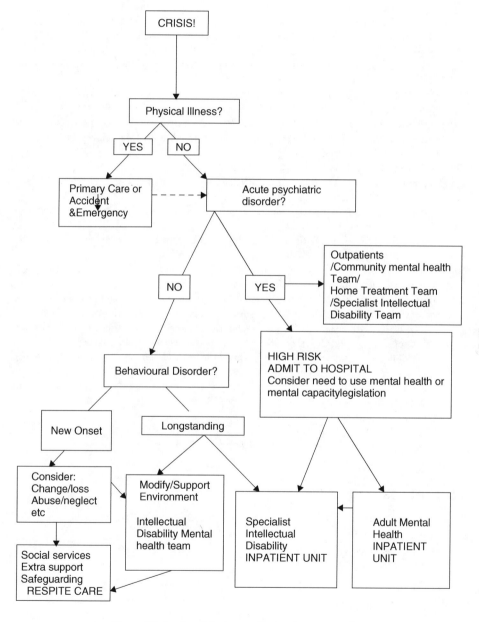

Figure 13.1   Possible care pathways in emergencies

References

1. Department of Health (2001) Valuing People–A National Strategy for Learning Disabilities for the 21st Century, Department of Health, London.
2. Department of Health (1999) A National Service Framework for Mental Health: Modern Standards and Service Models, Department of Health, London.
3. Smiley, E., Cooper, S.A., Finalxson, J. *et al.* (2007) Incidence and predictors of mental ill-health in adults with intellectual disabilities. *British Journal of Psychiatry*, **191**, 313–319.
4. Cooper, S.-A., Smiley, E., Morrison, J. *et al.* (2007) Mental ill health in adults with intellectual disabilities: prevalence and associated factors. *British Journal of Psychiatry*, **190**, 27–35.
5. Royal College of Psychiatrists (2001) *Diagnostic Criteria for Psychiatric Disorders for Use with Adults with Learning Disabilities/Mental Retardation (DC-LD)*, Gaskell Press, London.
6. Department of Health (2007) Services for People with Learning Disabilities and Challenging Behaviour or Mental Health Needs, (revised edition). (Mansell report), Department of Health, London.
7. Vanstralen M., Holt G.O. and Bouras N. (2003) Adults with learning disability and psychiatric problems, in *Seminars in the Psychiatry of Learning Disabilities*, 2nd edn (eds W. Fraser and M. Kerr), Gaskell Press, London.
8. Kerr, M. (2004) Improving the general health of people leaning disabilities. *Advances in Psychiatric Treatment*, **10**, 200–206.
9. Bradley, E. and Lofchy, J. (2005) Learning disability in the accident and emergency department. *Advances in Psychiatric Treatment*, **11**, 45–57.
10. Richards, M., Maughan, B., Hardy, R. *et al.* (2001) Long term affective disorder in people with mild learning disability. *British Journal of Psychiatry*, **179**, 523–527.
11. Merrick, J., Merrick, E., Lunsky, Y. *et al.* (2006) A review of suicidality in persons with intellectual disability. *Israel Journal of Psychiatry and Related Science*, **43** (4), 258–264.
12. A-Sheikh, A. and O'Hara, J. (2008) Psychiatric and mental state assessment in learning disabilities. *Advances in Mental Health and Learning Disabilities*, **2** (4), 21–28.
13. Royal College of Psychiatrists (1996) *Meeting the Mental Health Needs of People with Learning Disabilities*, Royal College of Psychiatrists, London.
14. Royal College of Psychiatrics (2003) Meeting the Mental Health Needs of people with Mild Learning Disability, Council Report CR 115, Royal College of Psychiatrists, London.
15. Hassiotis, A., Tyrer, P., and Oliver, P. (2003) Psychiatric assertive outreach and learning disability services. *Advances in Psychiatric Treatment*, **9**, 368–373.

Further reading

Fraser W. and Kerr D.M. (eds) (2003) *Seminars in the Psychiatry of Learning Disabilities*, 2nd edn, Gaskell Press, London.
Advances in Mental Health and Learning Disabilities (2008) **2** (4) (Whole issue).

14 Pharmacological Interventions

Department of Psychiatry, University of Birmingham, UK

14.1 Introduction

The general principles for using psychotropic medications for psychiatric disorders among adults with intellectual disabilities are similar to those used for the general population who do not have intellectual disabilities. No specific evidence base exists to recommend specific medications for psychiatric disorders among adults with intellectual disabilities, therefore in this chapter I will summarize the main points on pharmacological treatment of psychiatric disorders as suggested in the Maudsley guide [1] (see also the *Frith Prescribing Guidelines* [2]).

However, the primary aim of this chapter is to advise on the use of psychotropic medications for the management of problem behaviours among adults with intellectual disabilities because psychotropic medications are used outside their licensed indications for these problems, therefore good clinical practice is essential in this context.

Before starting any pharmacological treatment, the choice of medication should be discussed with the patients where possible and their carers, particularly the therapeutic effects, any adverse effects, discontinuation effects and alternative to medications. Clear advice should be given about how to contact professionals if needed out of hours. Accessible leaflets about the proposed medications are available and may be used for education, information and to aid adherence to treatment (see www.ld-medication.bham.ac.uk).

The health professionals seeking to commence treatment should always document the assessment of the capacity of the person to give informed consent to the proposed intervention. In the absence of capacity, as much as possible, a consensus

---

Intellectual Disability Psychiatry: a practical handbook   Angela Hassiotis, Diana Andrea Barron and Ian Hall (eds)
© 2009 John Wiley & Sons, Ltd

among the multidisciplinary team and the families/carers should be formed to decide which intervention is in the best interests of the person with intellectual disability. Sometimes a substitute decision maker is appointed on behalf of the person who does not have capacity.

14.2 Pharmacological treatment for mental disorders

Schizophrenia

Treatment with medication should be considered only as part of a comprehensive package of care. The National Institute for Health and Clinical Excellence (NICE; nice.org.uk) advises that new generation antipsychotic medications should be considered in the choice of first-line treatment. New generation antipsychotic medications (e.g. risperidone, olanzapine) should be considered for patients showing or reporting unacceptable adverse effects caused by old generation antipsychotic medications (e.g. haloperidol). Patients unresponsive to two different antipsychotic medications (one being a new generation) should be given clozapine. Depot antipsychotic medications should be used where there are grounds to suspect that a patient may be unlikely to adhere to prescribed oral therapy. New generation and old generation antipsychotic medications should not be prescribed together except during changeover of medication.

Acute mania or hypomania

Patients with no prior diagnosis of bipolar affective disorder should be started on antipsychotic medications (e.g. olanzapine, risperidone, quetiapine or conventional antipsychotic medications such as haloperidol). A patient with hypomania not receiving mood stabilizers should be started on sodium valproate (e.g. epilim chrono 500 mg/day or depakote 250 mg three times/day) or lithium (400 mg MR/day) or carbamazepine (200 mg MR twice/day). In patients with mania or mixed episodes a mood stabilizer should be added or the dose optimized and antipsychotic medications should be commenced. For all patients antidepressants should be withdrawn. As a second step benzodiazepine such as lorazepam up to 4 mg/day or clonazepam up to 2 mg/day may be added.

Bipolar disorders

For bipolar affective disorder mood stabilizers such as lithium or carbamazepine or sodium valproate or lamotrigine or topiramate could be used. For bipolar depression lithium alone or in combination with antidepressant medications or lamotrigine or a combination of olanzapine and fluoxetine can be used. For rapid cycling bipolar affective disorder, antidepressant medications should be withdrawn; possible precipitants such as alcohol, thyroid dysfunction and external stressors should be evaluated. Optimization of the treatment with mood stabilizers should include combination of medications though lithium may be less effective in this context. As a further step other medication options may be considered such as clozapine (usual dose), lamotrigine (up to 225 mg/day), levetiracetam (up to 200 mg/day), nimodipine (180 mg/day), olanzapine (usual dose), quetiapine (300–600 mg/day), risperidone (up to 6 mg/day) and thyroxine (150–200 mg/day) (in alphabetical order).

Depression

Antidepressants may be started and titrated to recognized therapeutic dose; their efficacy should be assessed over four to six weeks. If poorly tolerated, antidepressants from a different class can be prescribed. If ineffective, the dose should be increased and assessed over two weeks. If still ineffective, the diagnosis should be reconsidered and antidepressants from a different class may be prescribed. If still not effective, consider treatment for refractory depression including electroconvulsive therapy (ECT). If the patient responds to antidepressant medication, the treatment should be continued for six months to one year in case of first episode and longer in the case of patients who have had more than one episode of depression.

Generalized anxiety disorder (GAD)

Non-pharmacological interventions such as reassurance, anxiety management including relaxation training and cognitive behaviour therapy (CBT) should be tried first. For emergency management a short course of benzodiazepine for two to four weeks could be tried. For long-term psychotropic medications, selective serotonin reuptake inhibitors (SSRIs) (although may initially exacerbate symptoms, therefore a lower starting dose is often required or use in combination with a small dose of benzodiazepine initially) or venlafaxine (NICE recommends specialist referral) or a tricyclic antidepressant medication such as imipramine/clomipramine or pregabalin may be used. Other treatments include buspirone (has a delayed onset of action and low efficacy), hydroxizine, beta blockers (useful for somatic symptoms, particularly tachycardia; the evidence base for beta blockers' efficacy on anxiety symptoms is poor) and tiagabine.

Obsessive compulsive disorder (OCD)

Making a diagnosis of obsessive compulsive disorder (OCD) may be very difficult in adults with limited verbal skills and in those with autism as obsessions and compulsions may be confused with rituals that are a significant feature of autistic spectrum disorders.

However, in cases where OCD is ascertained, the primary interventions include psychological treatments such as exposure therapy, response prevention and other behaviour therapies such as CBT but a combined medication and psychological therapy may be most effective. Pharmacological options include SSRIs and clomipramine. Other medications to consider are antipsychotics such as risperidone or quetiapine but not haloperidol; also venlafaxine, buspirone, clomipramine, clonazepam (in general used to reduce associated anxiety) and mirtazapine augmentation of SSRIs.

Panic disorder

The primary treatment options are non-pharmacological such as CBT and anxiety management including relaxation training though a combined medication and psychological therapy may be most effective. In emergency a short-term use of benzodiazepine can be recommended. In the long term the options for psychotropic medications are SSRIs (therapeutic effect can be delayed and patients can experience an initial exacerbation of panic symptoms), some tricyclic antidepressants such as imipramine or clomipramine, and reboxetine. Other pharmacological options include monoamino-oxidase inhibitors (MAOIs), mirtazapine, sodium valproate and inositol.

Case vignette 14.1

A 62-year-old man with mild intellectual disabilities and a long-standing history of bipolar affective disorder was admitted to hospital with acute depression following several months of incapacity due to a hip replacement operation. He was tearful, sleeping poorly and being unresponsive. He reported paranoid delusions about having caused severe disturbance for which he believed he was hunted by the police.

He was recommenced on antipsychotic medication that he had stopped taking during his recuperation and lithium was added after a referral to neuropsychiatry. The latter was precipitated by findings of brain infarcts in the MRI. He recovered fully and was discharged home. He and his mother were informed about the side effects regarding lithium and the need for regular monitoring by his general practitioner. He was allocated to a community psychiatric nurse to assist with his health and medication who helped him to devise a health action plan.

Case vignette 14.2

A 45-year-old man with mild intellectual disabilities was referred with onset of depressive illness. It was precipitated by his partner's ill health and having been sacked from his job as a warehouse assistant. He was prescribed SSRIs and followed up for outpatient reviews. However, nine months into his treatment he became hyperactive and presented with lack of sleep, increased speech and inability to concentrate on any activities. The assessment indicated a manic episode likely due to the antidepressant which was stopped. He was started on antipsychotic medication and recovered fully. A community psychiatric nurse monitored his mental state.

14.3 Pharmacological management of problem behaviours among adults with intellectual disability

The rate of problem behaviours in adults with intellectual disabilities seems higher than the general population who do not have intellectual disabilities [3]. Management strategies for problem behaviours include both pharmacological and non-pharmacological interventions but in this chapter only pharmacological interventions will be discussed. The chapter will cover first some general principles which should underpin any intervention for problem behaviours and is based on the recently developed national guide on the use of psychotropic medication for the management of problem behaviours in adults with intellectual disabilities in the UK [4].

14.4 General principles underpinning the prescribing of medication

Assessment and formulation

The primary aim of management of problem behaviours in people with intellectual disabilities should be not to treat the behaviour per se but to identify and address the underlying cause of the behaviour. However, it is not always possible to find a cause for the problem behaviour. When this is the case, the management strategy should be to minimize the impact of the behaviour on the person, the environment around her/him and other people.

There may be many reasons for problem behaviours, including physical or mental health problems. Many factors internal to the person – such as negative childhood experiences, maladaptive coping strategies and so on, and external to the person – such as understimulating or overstimulating environment may contribute to problem behaviour. Sometimes behaviour may be used as a means of communication.

For example persons with severe intellectual disabilities who cannot speak or use a sign language may scream because they are in pain and they cannot communicate this message in any other way. Sometimes persons with intellectual disabilities may use behaviour to communicate their likes and dislikes.

Therefore, a thorough assessment of the causes of behaviour and their consequences, along with a formulation of personal, psychological, social, environmental, medical and psychiatric issues, is an absolute prerequisite in managing any problem behaviour. A proper assessment and formulation may need input from several disciplines and from families and carers. A multi-axial/multilayered diagnostic formulation (see DC-LD, UK; RCPsych and DM-ID, USA) [5, 6] may be useful in this context.

A formulation should be made even in the absence of a medical or psychiatric diagnosis. Box 14.1 summarizes the components of formulating a management plan of problem behaviours.

Box 14.1   Formulation of problem behaviours

- A list of the target problem behaviour(s) to be managed.

- A clear description of the problem behaviour, including frequency and severity.

- An assessment of the problem behaviour(s) and its causes.

- A differential diagnosis of causes giving rise to the problem behaviour.

- A record of reactions to and outcomes of the behaviour.

- An assessment of predisposing, precipitating and perpetuating risk factors.

- Consideration of all management options and their outcome.

- The rationale for the proposed management option.

- A risk assessment.

- Possible adverse effects from the proposed intervention(s).

- The likely effect of the proposed intervention(s) on the person's quality of life.

14.5 Input from the person with intellectual disabilities and their families and carers

A proper assessment and formulation will often depend on input from the person with intellectual disability and/or her/his family and carers. This input should continue at every stage of management. It is important to share information with the person with intellectual disability in a way that he or she can understand. This may require additional time and effort on the part of the health professionals and other members of the multidisciplinary team. It may also involve using innovative methods of information sharing, such as using pictures.

14.6 Multidisciplinary input

Multidisciplinary input may also be needed during implementation and monitoring of the management options. This may not always be possible to achieve because of lack of resources. Where relevant and if possible, an attempt should be made to secure multidisciplinary input to the process of managing problem behaviour.

When to consider medication

If there is an obvious medical or psychiatric cause for the behaviour, this should be managed in an appropriate way. If an underlying psychiatric disorder is treated with medication, the relevant guides governing the use of medication in the treatment of psychiatric disorders should be followed (see NICE, UK; www.nice.org.uk).

If no medical or psychiatric disorder can be recognized then non-pharmacological management should be considered depending on the formulation. Sometimes after considering other management options, medication may be used either on its own or as an adjunct to psychological interventions.

The exact situation under which pharmacological and psychological strategies should be implemented will depend on individual circumstances. However, it may be possible to improve the psychological well-being of the person by providing counselling and addressing social and environmental factors by finding more enjoyable activities to do during the day and using medication simultaneously to reduce anxiety. This strategy may be seen as an interim strategy, which then needs to be monitored carefully at regular intervals to assess its effectiveness. Box 14.2 summarizes the situations under which the clinicians may consider using medications.

Box 14.2   When to consider using pharmacological interventions

• Failure of non-medication-based interventions.

• Risk/evidence of harm/distress to self.

• Risk/evidence of harm/distress to others or property.

• High frequency/severity of problem behaviour.

• To treat an underlying psychiatric disorder or anxiety.

• To calm the person to enable implementation of non-medication-based interventions.

• Risk of breakdown to the person's placement.

• Good previous response to medication.

• Person/carer choice.

However, the lack of adequate or non-availability of psychological interventions should not be the reason for using medication but in practice this may happen. As much as possible this practice should be stopped or at least minimized and medication should be used for as short a period as possible.

Monitoring the effectiveness of the intervention

The effectiveness of any intervention and possible adverse effects should be monitored at regular intervals. This should include objective assessments with input from the person with intellectual disability and/or her/his family and carers, and members of other relevant disciplines, where necessary and possible. Examples of assessments include behavioural (both problem behaviour and other behaviours) and adverse effects, reports from families and carers, direct examination of physical and mental state, and if necessary relevant investigations such as blood tests, electrocardiogram (ECG) and other specialist investigations as needed.

An attempt should be made at each stage of monitoring to revisit and re-evaluate the formulation and the management plan. The aim is to prescribe medication, if necessary, at the lowest possible dose and for the minimum duration.

14.7 Prescribing within person centred planning

The management of behaviour should always be person centred. It should be influenced by the person her/himself and/or her/his carers and should be designed according to the person's best interests. The prescribing should not take place in isolation but should always be part of a much broader person centred care plan for the person with intellectual disability. In a person centred care plan, the person her/himself defines the important aspects of care in her/his own life.

14.8 Communication issues

The management plan should be communicated clearly to the person with intellectual disability and her/his family and carers. All other relevant professionals that are involved in the care of the person should be told about the management plan on a need-to-know basis. This process should be updated at regular intervals. Special care is needed and innovative approaches may be required when information about the management is shared with the person with intellectual disability and their family and carers.

Case vignette 14.3

K is a 60-year-old woman with moderate learning disabilities, autistic traits and a diagnosis of bipolar affective disorder. She was born in India and aged nine she came to live in the UK with her grandmother. Due to her grandmother's ill health K was then admitted to a long-stay hospital for people with learning disabilities, shortly after her arrival in London. She stayed there for 27 years and was eventually resettled to as part of the hospital's closure programme. She has been in supported housing since that time, with a two to one client to staff ratio and one member of staff sleeping in at night. She shares her flat with another female resident older than her. She can communicate verbally with

---

two- to three-word sentences; she is fully mobile, can attend to her self-care and can help with housework under supervision. Over the past few years K has experienced some physical health problems including mild heart failure, a hernia and bilateral ankle oedema. Despite the support, she has begun to shout and be restless at night but also during the day. Her activities have reduced as a result and she spends most of her time in the flat. The community intellectual disabilities team worked with the staff to explore how they worked with K and also observed K's behaviours and reviewed her treatment which consists of an antipsychotic and a mood stabilizer. A team of speech and language therapists, a psychiatrist and a psychologist alongside the home manager met weekly to finalize a support plan. This led to the implementation of relaxation strategies taught to staff in addition to multisensory sessions; demonstration of effective techniques to distract her attention and the investigation of her physical health. K has remained in her home and her problem behaviours have reduced. The multidisciplinary team will continue to meet at monthly intervals to review progress.

14.9 General principles for prescribing psychotropic medications

Anyone prescribing medication to manage problem behaviour in adults with intellectual disabilities should keep in mind the following points about good practice.

- Medication should be used only in the best interests of the person.

- All non-medication management options should have been considered and medication should be seen as necessary under the circumstances, or alongside non-medication management.

- Information about which interventions worked before and which did not should be noted.

- Relevant local and national protocols and guidelines should be followed.

- If previously interventions produced unacceptable adverse effects, the details should be noted.

- The effect of availability or non-availability of certain services and therapies on the treatment plan should be considered.

- If possible, evidence to show that the medication is cost-effective should be taken into account.

  Once the decision to prescribe is taken the clinician must:

- Ensure that a physical examination and appropriate investigations have been carried out.

- Ensure that the appropriate investigations such as blood tests, ECG and so on have been carried out at regular intervals and the results are available to the relevant professionals.

- Clarify to the person and/or her/his family or carers if the medication is being recommended outside its licensed indication. If this is the case, they should be told about the type and quality of evidence that is available to demonstrate its effectiveness.

- Identify a key person, usually a community psychiatric nurse, who will ensure that medication is administered appropriately and communicate all changes to the relevant parties.

- Provide the person and/or her/his family or carers with a copy of the agreed recommended treatment plan at the time of prescribing.

- Try to assess outcomes including adverse effects using both clinical opinion and standardized scales in order to monitor the severity and frequency of the target behaviour.

- Ensure arrangements for appropriate follow-up assessments have been made and that they take place.

- Ensure that one medication for the problem behaviour is prescribed at a time.

- Ensure that the medication should be used within the standard recommended dose range. Above the maximum recommended dose of medication should be used only in exceptional circumstances after full discussion with all the relevant stakeholders under appropriate safeguards and regular reviews.

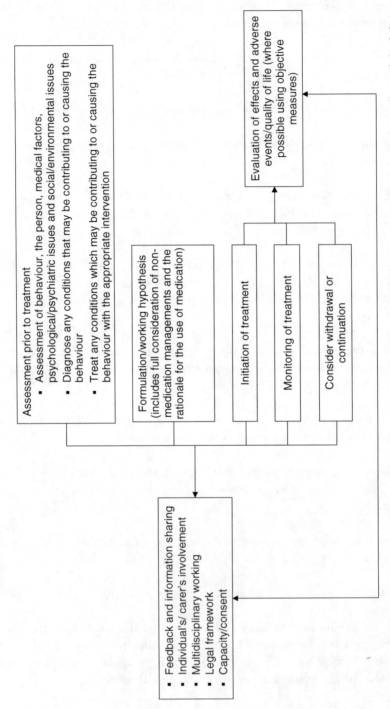

Figure 14.1 Key processes associated with using medication to manage problem behaviour in adults with intellectual disabilities

Assessment prior to treatment
- Assessment of behaviour, the person, medical factors, psychological/psychiatric issues and social/environmental issues
- Diagnose any conditions that may be contributing to or causing the behaviour
- Treat any conditions which may be contributing to or causing the behaviour with the appropriate intervention

Formulation/working hypothesis (includes full consideration of non-medication managements and the rationale for the use of medication)

Initiation of treatment

Monitoring of treatment

Consider withdrawal or continuation

Evaluation of effects and adverse events/quality of life (where possible using objective measures)

- Feedback and information sharing
- Individual's/ carer's involvement
- Multidisciplinary working
- Legal framework
- Capacity/consent

- Start with a low dose and titrate the dose up slowly.

- Use medication at the lowest required dose for the minimum period of time necessary.

- Consider the withdrawing of medication and explore non-medication management options at all times.

Figure 14.1 summarizes the main points of prescribing medication in adults with intellectual disabilities and challenging behaviour.

14.10 Evidence of the risks associated with prescribing medication in adults with intellectual disabilities and problem behaviour

Most medications carry a potential risk associated with adverse events. However, evidence is largely gathered from studies among patients with psychoses who do not have intellectual disabilities. For example, current evidence shows that new generation antipsychotic medications carry a certain amount of risk relating to weight gain, cardiac abnormalities and various metabolic abnormalities, including impaired glucose tolerance, lipid metabolism and prolactin metabolism.

There is lack of high quality evidence to either support or refute concerns that people with intellectual disabilities may be at greater risk of the adverse effects of medication than people from the general population who do not have intellectual disabilities.

The shortage of such evidence does not mean that medication is associated with an unacceptable risk specifically for adults with intellectual disabilities.

In view of the above, the following general points should be kept in mind.

Adverse events

- Discuss with the person and/or her/his family and carers common and serious adverse events related to the treatment (where possible provide accessible information in writing).

- Also advise what action to take if a serious adverse event takes place.

- All adverse events should be recorded properly.

Choice of medication

It is not possible to recommend currently specific medication for the treatment of specific problem behaviour because there is no evidence to support such recommendations. However, Appendix 14.A provides a list of medications that are used for the management of problem behaviour in adults with intellectual disabilities with their common adverse effects (also see Unwin and Deb for a consensus survey in the UK [7]).

Discontinuation of treatment

- Once a medication is prescribed, the risk−benefit profile should continue to be evaluated regularly, with particular emphasis on the person's and her/his family and carers' quality of life.

- Consideration of a reduction in the dose or withdrawing the medication and exploring non-medication management options should be ongoing.

14.11 In instances where the behaviour re-emerges after reducing the dose or withdrawing the medication

- There should be a relapse management plan in place when considering medication withdrawal (see Figure 14.2).

- Be aware of the withdrawal effect of certain medication and allow adequate time for that to settle before reconsidering the use of medication.

- Always consider non-medication-based interventions and reassess the initial formulation and rationale for using the medication.

14.12 Poly-prescribing

It is not uncommon for people with intellectual disabilities to take medication for a wide variety of disorders and illnesses. However, the term poly-prescribing in this document is used to describe the prescribing of more than one medication for a particular indication, in this case problem behaviour.

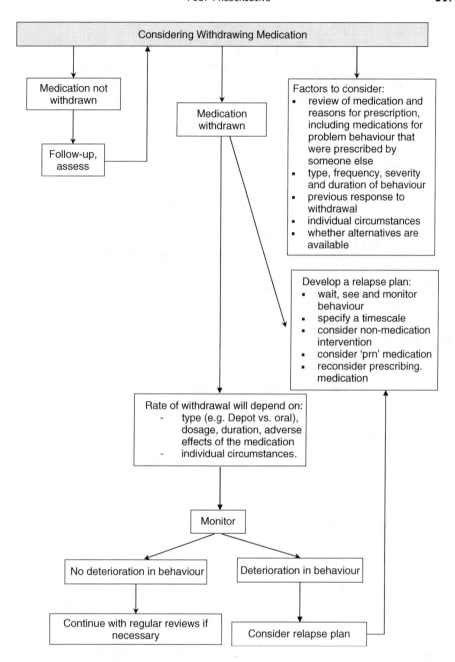

Figure 14.2 Flow chart for withdrawal of medication

Evidence to support poly-prescribing

There is a lack of studies of combinations of psychotropic medications to manage problem behaviour among adults with intellectual disabilities. However, the evidence based on observational studies suggests that the reduction in poly-prescribing not only improves behaviour but also the quality of life of the person for whom medication is prescribed.

Therefore if an add-on medication is indicated, the following points should be kept in mind

- If the add-on medication is ineffective, reassess the situation.

- If the first medication is to be continued, the reasons for continuing to use more than one medication simultaneously for the same indication must be recorded.

- The use of an add-on medication from the same medication category is not advisable (the exception is anti-epileptic medications for the treatment of epilepsy).

- If the combination is effective, try to withdraw or at least reduce the dose of one of the medications at a future date.

- Always consider the option of either a non-medication intervention or using such an intervention in combination with the medication.

- Try to return to monotherapy as soon as possible.

- Avoid using more than two medications simultaneously for the same indication.

- More than two medications should be used only under exceptional circumstances.

- Try to secure another clinician's opinion if more than two medications are to be used simultaneously.

- The use of more than three medications simultaneously is difficult to justify unless they are used for other indications, such as simultaneous epilepsy or psychiatric disorder.

Evidence to support withdrawing medication that has been prescribed for a long period

Studies of withdrawing medication show that, in a proportion of cases, the medication can be successfully withdrawn after a long period of use [8, 9]. In a proportion of cases, the dose can be reduced, although total withdrawal is not possible, and in some cases, it is difficult to even reduce the dose of medication after a long period of use. Many factors affect the success of withdrawal of medication, including non-medical factors such as the training and the attitude of care staff. However, on the basis of such evidence it is not possible to recommend which medication to withdraw and how. Box 14.3 summarizes general recommendations to be followed up in such cases.

Box 14.3 The person on one or more medications for a long period of time to manage problem behaviour

- Try to stabilize the person's problem behaviour on a minimum number of medications prescribed at the lowest possible dose, or no medication.

- Follow the recommendations given in the 'Discontinuation of treatment' section of this chapter.

- Withdraw one medication at a time.

- Withdraw medication slowly.

- If necessary, allow time (sometimes a few weeks) after withdrawing one medication and before starting to withdraw another.

Appendix 14.A Commonly used psychotropic medications, their dosage, adverse effects and necessary investigations

Antipsychotic medications

Commonly used *old generation antipsychotic medications* are chlorpromazine (more sedating), haloperidol (more extrapyramidal adverse effects), thioridazine (restricted use in the UK).

- **Possible adverse effects:** are extrapyramidal symptoms such as acute dystonia (acute opisthotonous-arching of body backwards), Parkinsonian symptoms (tremor, stiffness, etc.), akathisia (external and internal restlessness), dystonia (slow abnormal movement) and tardive dyskinesia (TD; long-term adverse effect; abnormal movements starting with oro-facial muscles but may also affect limbs and shoulders). Also dry mouth, blurred vision and constipation. Other adverse effects are cardiac and sexual dysfunction, and metabolic effects such as raised prolactin level. Serious adverse effect is neuroleptic malignant syndrome (NMS; primarily autonomic disturbance such as high temperature, high blood pressure, muscle stiffness; confirmatory investigation includes raised muscle CPK level; treatment involves immediate withdrawal of antipsychotics and symptomatic treatment).

- **New generation antipsychotic medications:** are risperidone, olanzapine, quetiapine, clozapine, aripiprazole, piperidone, amisulpride, zotepine and sertindole (restricted use in the UK). These drugs affect D2/4, 5HT, also alpha, H1, histamine receptors and so on.

- **Possible adverse effects:** are extrapyramidal symptoms, NMS, metabolic syndrome, such as glucose intolerance (leading to diabetes mellitus), hyperprolactinaemia, hyperlipidaemia and weight gain. Other adverse effects are drowsiness, agranulocytosis (particularly associated with clozapine), cardiac arrhythmia (prolonged QT interval) and sexual dysfunction. Most antipsychotics are epileptogenic (clozapine in high doses is particularly bad for this) but new generations are probably slightly better than the old generations in this respect.

- **Common investigation necessary:** for these medications are BP, weight, full blood count (FBC), liver function test (LFT), renal function test (RFT), serum electrolytes, lipid profile, blood glucose, ECG, serum prolactin level and so on.

Antidepressant medications

- **Old generation:** of tricyclic antidepressants are amitriptyline, clomipramine, imipramine and so on.

- **Possible adverse effects:** are dry mouth, constipation, blurred vision, hypotension (cholinergic adverse effects), cardiac failure and fatality associated with overdose.

- **Common investigations necessary:** for prescribing these medications are FBC, RFT, U&Es, LFT and ECG.

- **New generation:** antidepressants are SSRIs such as fluoxetine, fluvoxamine, sertraline, citalopram, escitalopram, paroxetine, venlafaxine, which is a serotonin and nor-adrenaline reuptake inhibitor (SNRI). Others are duloxetine, flupentixol, mirtazapine, reboxetine and tryptophan.

- **Possible adverse effects:** of these medications are agitation, sleep problem, sexual dysfunction, withdrawal problem, serotonin syndrome (associated with SSRIs), increased risk of suicidal ideas.

- **Common investigations necessary:** are FBC, LFT, RFT, U&Es and ECG (for venlafaxine).

Mood stabilizers

Lithium

- **Possible adverse effects:** are tremor, renal failure, thyroid dysfunction, confusion in toxicity.

- **Common investigations necessary:** are serum lithium level (in order to adjust the dose and detect toxicity), FBC, RFT, U&Es and thyroid function test (TFT). Pre-lithium work-up should include ECG, TFT, RFT (serum creatinine and urea) and U&Es.

Anti-epileptic medications

Carbamazepine

- **Possible adverse effects:** are drowsiness, double vision, ataxia, hyponatraemia and skin rash (may lead to Stevens-Johnson syndrome).

- **Investigations necessary:** are FBC, LFT, serum electrolytes and RFT.

Sodium valproate (valproic acid/semisodium valproate)

- **Possible adverse effects:** are drowsiness, weight gain, hair loss, skin rash, ataxia and liver function failure in rare cases. Teratogenecity should be kept in mind if used in women of childbearing age.

- **Investigations necessary:** are FBC, LFT, U&Es and RFT.

Beta blockers

Atenolol and propranolol in high doses as well as anti-anxiety drugs such as diazepam have been used for problem behaviour. The use of benzodiazepine such as the diazepam is restricted for short period of use (four to six weeks). Opioid antagonists such as naloxone (intramuscular or intravenous preparations) and naltrexone (oral preparations) have been used particularly to treat severe self-injurious behaviour (SIB). However, evidence for their efficacy is equivocal (see www.ld-medication. bham.ac.uk).

References

1. Taylor, D., Paton, C. and Kerwin, R. (2007) *The Maudsley Prescribing Guidelines*, Taylor & Francis, London.
2. Bhaumik S. and Branford D. (eds) (2008) *The Frith Prescribing Guidelines: For Adults with Intellectual Disability*, HealthComm UK Ltd, Aberdeen.
3. Deb, S., Thomas, M. and Bright, C. (2001) Mental disorder in adults with intellectual disability. 2: the rate of behaviour disorders among a community-based population aged between 16–64 years. *Journal of Intellectual Disability Research*, **45** (6), 506–514.
4. Deb, S., Clarke, D. and Unwin, G. (2006) *Using Medication to Manage Behaviour Problems Among Adults with a Learning Disability: Quick Reference Guide (QRG)*, University of Birmingham, MENCAP, The Royal College of Psychiatrists, London, ISBN 0855370947. www.ld-medication.bham.ac.uk.
5. Royal College of Psychiatrists (RCPsych) (2001) *DC-LD: Diagnostic Criteria for Psychiatric Disorders for Use with Adults with Learning Disabilities/Mental Retardation*, Occasional Paper OP48, Gaskell Press, London.
6. Fletcher R., Loschen E., Stavrakaki C., and First M. (eds) (2007) *Diagnostic Manual-Intellectual Disability (DM-ID): A Textbook of Diagnosis of Mental Disorders in Persons with Intellectual Disability*, The National Association for the Dually Diagnosed (NADD) Press and the American Psychiatric Association (APA), Washington, DC.
7. Unwin, G. and Deb, S. (2008) Use of medication for the management of behaviour problems among adults with intellectual disabilities: a clinicians' consensus survey. *American Journal on Mental Retardation*, **113** (1), 19–31.
8. Ahmed, Z., Fraser, W., Kerr, M.P. *et al.* (2000) Reducing antipsychotic medication in people with a learning disability. *The British Journal of Psychiatry*, **178**, 42–46.
9. Branford, D. (1996) Factors associated with the successful or unsuccessful withdrawal of antipsychotic drug therapy prescribed for people with learning disabilities. *Journal of Intellectual Disability Research*, **40**, 322–329.

Further reading

National Institute of Clinical Excellence. www.nice.org.uk.
Psychotropic medication leaflets accessible version: www.ld-medication.bham.ac.uk.

15 Psychological Interventions

Katrina Scior
Research Department of Clinical, Educational & Health Psychology, University College London, UK

15.1 Introduction

For a long time the main role of psychology within intellectual disability services was the provision of psychological testing and treatment through the application of social learning theory. This was offered particularly in the form of behaviour therapy to manage behaviours deemed undesirable in the large institutions and to teach new skills. Historically the emotional lives of people with intellectual disabilities were largely neglected. Some have argued that such neglect arose from the general disdain with which this client group has been treated [1, 2]. An alternative explanation is that in the era of institutionalization the physical conditions of people's lives were so impoverished that improving these had to take precedence over addressing their emotional needs.

With the gradual closure of long-stay institutions and an increased focus on community care, support to manage individuals' moves into the community became a significant aspect of psychological work, as did an array of other activities aimed at increasing quality of life. Since the early 1990s there has been an increased focus on the emotional and mental health needs of people with intellectual disabilities and a steady development of therapeutic work. The role of psychology within intellectual disability services has expanded and diversified enormously as a result. Where, once, only behavioural approaches were on offer, in many services now a whole range of psychological interventions is available. These may be delivered either directly with the person with intellectual disabilities or through indirect work, such as with a staff

Intellectual Disability Psychiatry: a practical handbook   Angela Hassiotis, Diana Andrea Barron and Ian Hall (eds)
© 2009 John Wiley & Sons, Ltd

team or the management of an organization, or a combination of both modes of delivery. Furthermore in line with their training as scientist-practitioners, psychologists have an important role in designing and completing research and service evaluation.

All psychological interventions are (or certainly should be) based on a thorough assessment and formulation which pays close attention to the context of the person's life and their presenting problems. Depending on the theoretical model guiding assessment, this may focus more on:

- current emotional functioning and its roots in early development

- a detailed understanding of events

- cognitions and

- behavioural patterns in the here and now

- or relational issues.

The scientist-practitioner model underlying clinical psychology is guided by a formulation of the presenting problem which makes sense of the information gained during assessment and draws on psychological theory to provide an understanding how the problem developed and what factors may be maintaining it. This formulation will then guide the planning of any intervention and will be revised as additional or contradictory information emerges. Finally, the outcomes of any intervention should be assessed using valid and reliable methods.

15.2 Frameworks for psychological work

Prior to considering psychological interventions in detail, it will be useful for the reader to be familiar with some broad frameworks which guide the practice of clinical psychologists. A prominent one notes that all psychological work with people with intellectual disabilities should be socially valid and person centred [3]. Thus it should address socially significant problems, in a manner acceptable to those involved *and* to non-disabled people and result in socially meaningful and important outcomes, while keeping the person at the centre of support.

A further important framework for clinical psychologists is attention to risk and protective factors. These fall broadly into four domains, namely biological, psychological, social and environmental. The efforts of clinical psychologists are largely focused on understanding and tackling problems in the last three domains which may give rise to current difficulties. Psychological risk factors common to many people with intellectual disabilities include:

- a history of unstable attachments

- learned helplessness

- low self-esteem

- limited social skills and

- poor problem solving skills.

Social and environmental risk factors relate to social barriers and dependence on support from carers, and may include:

- stigmatization and segregation

- over-protection

- lack of opportunities

- experiences of neglect and abuse

- deprivation and poverty

- limited social networks and

- poorly managed changes and losses.

Which of these are targeted for an intervention depends as much on the psychological formulation of the presenting problem, as it does on resources and the particular theoretical model the clinician draws on.

15.3 Overview of main psychological approaches

At risk of oversimplifying the multifaceted role of psychology in intellectual disability services, this section will provide a summary of the main approaches used within this context.

Table 15.1 Main psychological interventions

- Behaviour therapy and functional analysis
- Cognitive behaviour therapy
- Psychodynamic therapy
- Systemic therapy
- Indirect work/consultation with organizations drawing on any of the above models
- Provision of training for carers.

The reader is referred to a number of comparative reviews that consider several of these approaches [4–6]. For the purposes of this chapter each approach will be outlined and briefly discussed. Of note, psychological theories have informed the development of other interventions, for example interventions designed to target ASDs or aimed at increasing engagement levels for people with the most severe disabilities and associated communication difficulties (intensive interaction). However, such interventions are mostly carried out by carers and support workers, not by psychologists. This chapter will focus on interventions typically carried out by clinical psychologists.

It is important to acknowledge the contrast between routes into help taken by most persons with intellectual disabilities and one of the prominent definitions of psychotherapy, namely as 'an interpersonal process designed to bring about modifications of feelings, cognitions, attitudes and behaviour which have proved troublesome to the person seeking help from a trained professional' [7]. In the case of people with intellectual disabilities, frequently the person concerned will not be the one seeking help, and indeed may at least at first sight not appear to be particularly troubled. Clinicians should carefully bear this in mind when considering how to respond to any request for help, and deciding on the most appropriate locus for intervention (rather than assuming *a priori* that this should be the person with intellectual disabilities).

A number of therapeutic orientations popular within mainstream psychotherapy, most notably interpersonal, cognitive analytic and existential therapy, will not be considered here as to date they have found no or limited documented application in the area of intellectual disabilities.

15.4 Behaviour therapy

Some of the most important and lasting applications of behavioural theory and particularly operant conditioning principles are in the area of challenging behaviour.

Functional analysis, the attempt to understand the meaning or underlying functions of a behaviour, and positive behavioural support have been considered in Chapter 9 on challenging behaviour and shall not be discussed further here. It is worth reiterating though that functional analysis should be the approach of choice where challenging behaviour is severe and the most urgent target for intervention, as the evidence base supports its use in such instances [8]. Therefore unless services have specialist challenging behaviour teams, it would be unusual not to consider involving psychology in such cases. Readers are advised to consult the joint guidelines issued by the Royal College of Psychiatry, British Psychological Society and the Royal College of Speech and Language Therapists [8], which offer in-depth guidance on assessment and intervention in this area.

Interventions based on the principles of social learning theory and applied behavioural analysis inform many other psychological interventions offered in intellectual disability services. Other forms of therapy, particularly cognitive behaviour therapy (CBT) and to a lesser extent systemic therapy, may draw on behavioural components as an integral part of, or add-on to, the intervention.

15.5 Cognitive behaviour therapy

CBT has become very influential in the mental health field, not least due to its strong evidence base. Over recent years there has been a marked increase in the use of this approach with people with intellectual disabilities.

Although a wide range of interventions fall under the umbrella of CBT, they all share these common features:

- A combination of behavioural and cognitive components.

- An assumption that cognitive processes affect emotion as well as behaviour and vice versa.

- An assumption that psychological difficulties are the result of maladaptive cognitive processes, for example dysfunctional core beliefs, a tendency to overgeneralize or reach overly negative conclusions and that behaviours reinforce these cognitions.

- A belief that these processes may well be understandable in terms of the person's experiences, yet prove unhelpful in the here and now.

The aim of CBT is to challenge and bring about change by generating new and more adaptive ways of thinking alongside learning more adaptive ways of behaving.

Table 15.2 Key assumptions made in CBT

Clients show some capacity for:

- Abstract reasoning
- Generalization
- Socio-emotional understanding
- Verbal communication
- Establishing a collaborative relationship
- Sense of agency
- Motivation to change and preparedness for therapy.

This approach is now the treatment of choice for anxiety disorders and depression in the general adult population, due to convincing evidence of its effectiveness [9]. With people with intellectual disabilities CBT has been used and evaluated in the treatment of a broad range of conditions including anxiety disorders, depression, social skills deficits, symptoms of psychosis and anger management [10–14].

Of note, CBT makes a number of assumptions which are highly relevant to considering the suitability of this approach for people with intellectual disabilities.

Some of the difficulties commonly associated with intellectual disabilities mean that CBT may either not be suitable for certain individuals or will need substantial adaptations. Such difficulties may be present mainly at the individual level, including problems with abstract reasoning, generalization and verbal communication. Others operate at the social level; a history of negative experiences of being stigmatized and having little control over one's life may render establishing a collaborative relationship and exercising control and agency in working towards personal change particularly challenging.

In order to engage in and benefit from CBT clients need to show at least a basic capacity to recognize and name emotions, and link emotions and beliefs to events. A number of authors have suggested ways of assessing the suitability of CBT for a given client [15, 16]. Language ability appears to be significantly associated with the skills implicated in CBT and performance on the British Picture Vocabulary Scales has been suggested as a good predictor of such skills [16].

Clinical reports almost invariably acknowledge the need to adapt standard CBT to meet the needs of this client group. Key adaptations include increasing the number of sessions, simplifying language and tasks, liberal use of repetition and rehearsal and involving others close to the person. Adaptation to techniques may include drawings and pictures to set an agenda and develop a shared formulation, the use of pictures and role plays to access thoughts and feelings and simplified homework tasks.

Case vignette 15.1.1   Samantha

Samantha, a 21-year-old white British woman with mild learning disabilities, is referred by her parents. Samantha is the youngest of three sisters. She lives with her parents; both her sisters have left home to attend university. Samantha attended mainstream schools but says once she was in her teens she found this more and more of a struggle. She had few friends at school. Her best friend Bessy moved away to the country when Samantha was 14. Samantha left school without passing any of her GCSEs and moved onto a life skills course at the local college. Since this came to an end 18 months ago, Samantha has mostly stayed at home.

Her parents are concerned that Samantha frequently appears tearful and they have overheard her saying. 'It's no point. I wish I was dead.' They contact the team and ask for help with Samantha's depression.

The approach a CBT therapist might follow in trying to help Samantha and her family is outlined in Case vignette 15.1.2.

Case vignette 15.1.2   Samantha: a CBT approach

A CBT therapist would focus on Samantha's thoughts and beliefs which give rise to her low mood, and the behaviours maintaining these. The therapist might discover that Samantha has always negatively compared herself to her sisters and holds a core belief that she is unlovable and will fail at anything she tries. Accordingly she avoids new challenges and social contacts. Therapeutic work would focus on collecting evidence which contradicts Samantha's overly negative picture of herself and her place in the world and her tendency for black and white thinking. Behavioural work might encourage her to try new activities in a controlled manner and to evaluate these in therapy sessions, with the aim of shifting her cognitions.

Overall the therapist might see Samantha for 16 individual weekly sessions, and invite her parents to regular reviews with Samantha to evaluate her progress and engage her parents in supporting the therapy.

15.6 Psychodynamic therapy

The central aim in psychodynamic therapy is to help the client identify and understand what is happening in their inner world, in the context of their personal history.

By trying to bring unconscious processes into greater consciousness, psychodynamic therapy aims to alleviate some of the distress associated with unresolved feelings. This is done primarily through the use of interpretation of the client's behaviour and verbalizations during sessions. The emotional experience associated with the therapist tolerating thoughts and feelings which the client previously deemed intolerable is an important element of psychodynamic therapy [9]. One might argue it is of prime importance for people with intellectual disabilities who may have had few prior opportunities to express negative emotions in the context of a trusting relationship.

A number of practitioners have written about the use of psychodynamic theory to understand the inner lives of people with intellectual disabilities [1, 17–19]. Some of their key advances include drawing attention to the importance of the need to come to terms with the disability itself; 'secondary handicap', the process whereby primary impairments are exaggerated to defend against painful feelings of being different [1–19] and overwhelming fears of others' unconscious death wishes [19]. Psychodynamic therapy has been provided to address the after-effects of trauma and loss, fears and other negative emotions which may often be held at an unconscious level by people with intellectual disabilities.

Attention to the *transference* and *counter-transference*, the process of making conscious what the client may be feeling by the therapist carefully observing their own reactions, is of great importance when working with people with intellectual disabilities, as they are less likely to be able to identify or verbalize their emotions [20]. Therapists must allow enough time for this work, as it may take considerable time to reach core difficulties and a premature end to treatment may leave the client exposed and with a reduced capacity to defend against their negative effects.

The approach a psychodynamic therapist might follow in trying to help Samantha is outlined in Case vignette 15.1.3.

Case vignette 15.1.3   The case of Samantha revisited – a psychodynamic approach

Rather than asking lots of assessment-style questions, the therapist would let Samantha lead the session. In noticing that Samantha would avoid making eye contact and generally appear reluctant to talk, the therapist might wonder aloud whether Samantha was finding it difficult being with her, and that she might not quite believe that the therapist would want to know her. This might allow Samantha to express some of the very negative feelings she held towards herself, perhaps by saying, 'Yes, why would you want to know me? I'm useless.'

During subsequent sessions Samantha might frequently talk about her sisters and their successes and get upset. At these times the therapist might notice that she experienced intense feelings of anger towards Samantha's parents for leaving

> Samantha to feel left behind. She would make gentle links between Samantha's experiences and her apparent anger towards her parents, which felt intolerable to Samantha and hence had become directed at her sisters and herself.

Beail and colleagues have tried to demonstrate the effectiveness of this approach with people with intellectual disabilities [21, 22]. They have shown that psychodynamic treatment can lead to reductions in symptomatology and increase the individual's capacity to assimilate problematic experiences [23].

15.7 Systemic therapy

The term 'systemic' is wide ranging and does not have one set definition, yet all approaches under the systemic umbrella start from the fundamental assumption that the system that gives rise to a problem is the most appropriate focus for intervention, rather than symptoms or increased insight. A systems approach views the person with intellectual disabilities as part of a dynamic, interactive and interdependent system which includes the family and wider social system. Unlike in a linear model of causation, in systems theory something that happens to one member of the system will affect all other members of the system [24]. As such, the main focus in systemic work is on the system of which the identified person is part, particularly on the relationships and interactions between people in the system. In the case of adults with intellectual disabilities, the system in focus may well be the family, but frequently it is the wider system the person interacts with, such as care providers and their organizations.

It has been argued that a systems approach is particularly well suited to this client group, who tend to live with their families or in groups of non-related adults and who are likely to find their life paths strongly influenced by others' views and actions [25]. Its focus on context, communication and multiple perspectives has been described as holding great promise when faced with the often complex systems and relationships which individuals with intellectual disabilities are part of [26]. Early reports of systemic therapy with this client group drew on similar themes as the psychodynamic literature of the time, namely trauma, loss and grief, yet aimed for change by working with the whole family, rather than the referred individual [27, 28]. More recently systems theory has been used in an intellectual disability context to get away from a focus on difference and pathology, instead aiming to refocus the system's attention on strengths, resources and abilities that may well be overlooked. In addition, an analysis of the social and cultural context and attention to differences in power and opportunities are integral to current, postmodern systemic developments [26]. This focus places such work closely in line with current policies which emphasize choice and empowerment [29]. Systemic therapy may be offered to the individual and members of their family. Others have used a systemic approach to work with staff teams and their organizations, for example to reconsider the support system's view of the person and the perceived problem.

Case vignette 15.1.4   Samantha's story revisited – a systemic approach

In responding to her parents' and Samantha's concerns, a systemic therapist would be most interested in the relationships between Samantha and those close to her which gave rise to and maintain the negative stories she tells about herself. The therapist would aim to hear the perspectives of others, whether present in therapy sessions or not. Questions, for example what Samantha's sisters and her friend Bessy would say about Samantha and value about her might bring forth positive qualities and resources which have become forgotten. Her parents might recognize that they have been much more protective of Samantha than her sisters, because she is their youngest and because they view her as much more vulnerable. Such conversations in therapy may help Samantha to discover how much she is loved, and her parents might decide to support Samantha in trying new activities and ways of making new friends, as their previous protective stance was guided by their intense love of their daughter but ultimately disabled her further.

A consistent theme in the systemic literature is how to ensure that the individual with intellectual disabilities is fully involved and ensuring that the person's voice is heard. However, it is important to respect established patterns of conversation and avoid over-inviting the individual in families where others customarily talk for the person, as this may silence others; instead change needs to happen in small steps [30].

To date, however, the evidence base for this approach with people with intellectual disabilities is very limited. This is not least because many systemic therapists feel that the 'evidence-based treatment' paradigm and associated methods of evidence production have a poor fit with a model which tries to get away from focussing on symptoms and which views clients as the experts on their lives and therapy very much as a shared endeavour rather than something that is 'done to' clients. The approach a systemic therapist might follow in trying to help Samantha and her family is outlined in Case vignette 15.1.4.

15.8 Work at the organizational level

Much of psychological work is not undertaken with an individual client in the therapy room, but instead involves the application of psychological theory in working with an organization. One popular mode of delivery, namely consultation to an organization, can be informed by any of the main psychological models. The potential value of a consultation mode may be particularly indicated where similar and perhaps recurring concerns seem to be expressed about several service users, or where past attempts at change have been hampered by organizational obstacles. In such instances psychologists may decide that work with the management of an organization or a whole staff team is more likely to result in positive change, for example by changing patterns of interaction, increasing empathy and understanding or arriving at more consistent support practices.

Psychologists in many services have an important role in providing training, usually for support staff. This mostly takes the form of psycho-education and may aim at achieving changes in knowledge, attitudes and behaviour.

15.9 Evidence for psychological interventions

Research evaluating the outcomes of psychological interventions with people with intellectual disabilities, other than those derived from behavioural theory, is still very limited. Randomized controlled trials (RCTs) on any of the interventions covered in this chapter are non-existent and concerns have repeatedly been expressed about the viability of RCTs with this population. Obstacles to the production of an evidence base include potential difficulties obtaining informed consent (and research ethical approval for a population deemed by many 'highly vulnerable'), ethical concerns regarding control-group designs which involve a no treatment condition, the increased study period due to the longer time needed for change and small sample sizes [31]. Therefore the majority of evidence consists of single case studies, although there have been some recent efforts at producing practice-based evidence by joining forces across clinical services [22, 32].

15.10 Conclusions

This chapter has provided an overview of the wide range of psychological interventions which may be available to people with learning disabilities and those close to them. Evidence is slowly beginning to emerge demonstrating the effectiveness of some of these approaches with people with intellectual disabilities. However, the availability of the interventions considered and the competence with which they are executed can be highly variable. Furthermore clinicians' perceptions of their own competence in a particular therapeutic approach and the level of the client's functioning appear to be important factors in influencing the provision of psychological therapy to people with intellectual disabilities [33]. Of note, at a time dominated by discussions about evidence based practice, the same study found that the perceived effectiveness of any therapy with this population appeared somewhat less important in guiding treatment decisions, although this may relate at least partly to the limited evidence base on which clinicians base these.

What is offered may be a combination of several of the approaches outlined in this chapter either in parallel, sequence or to complement interventions offered by other disciplines. Due to the complex nature of the needs of many clients, provision of a discreet psychological intervention is the exception rather than the rule. Change will often be much slower than in any textbook descriptions of the approach or in manualied treatments and may require significant adaptations to ensure that they are person centred and likely to result in meaningful positive change.

References

1. Sinason, V. (1992) *Mental Handicap and the Human Condition: New Approaches from the Tavistock*, Free Association Books, London.
2. Bender, M. (1993) The unoffered chair: the history of therapeutic disdain towards people with a learning disability. *Clinical Psychology Forum*, **54**, 7–12.
3. Emerson E., Hatton C., Bromley J. and Caine A. (eds) (1998) *Clinical Psychology and People with Intellectual Disabilities*, John Wiley & Sons, Chichester.
4. Beail, N. (2003) What works for people with mental retardation? Critical commentary on cognitive-behavioural and psychodynamic psychotherapy research. *Mental Retardation*, **41**, 468–472.
5. Whitehouse, R., Tudway, J., Look, R. and Kroese, B. (2006) Adapting individual psychotherapy for adults with intellectual disabilities: a comparative review of the cognitive-behavioural and psychodynamic literature. *Journal of Applied Research in Intellectual Disabilities*, **19**, 55–65.
6. Willner, P. (2005) The effectiveness of psychotherapeutic interventions for people with learning disabilities: a critical overview. *Journal of Intellectual Disability Research*, **49**, 73–85.
7. Strupp H.H. (1978) Psychotherapy research and practice: an overview, in *Handbook of Psychotherapy and Behaviour Change: An Empirical Analysis*, 2nd edn (eds S.L. Garfield and A.C. Bergin), John Wiley & Sons, Inc., New York, pp. 3–22.
8. Banks, R., Bush, A., Baker, P. *et al.* (2007) Challenging Behaviour: A Unified Approach, Royal College of Psychiatrists, British Psychological Society and Royal College of Speech and Language Therapists, London, CR 144. Available at: http://www.rcpsych.ac.uk/files/pdfversion/cr144.pdf.
9. Roth, A. and Fonagy, P. (2005) *What Works for Whom? A Critical Review of Psychotherapy Research*, 2nd edn, Guilford, New York.
10. Dagnan, D. and Jahoda, A. (2006) Cognitive-behavioural intervention for people with intellectual disability and anxiety disorders. *Journal of Applied Research in Intellectual Disabilities*, **19**, 91–97.
11. Hassiotis, A. and Hall, I. (2008) Behavioural and cognitive-behavioural interventions in the treatment of outwardly directed aggression in people with a learning disability (Revised review). *Cochrane Database of Systematic Reviews* 3.

12. Kroese B., Dagnan D. and Loumidis K. (eds) (1997) *Cognitive-behaviour Therapy for People with Learning Disabilities*, Routledge, London.
13. Lindsay, W.R. (1999) Cognitive therapy. *The Psychologist*, **12**, 238–241.
14. Taylor, J.L. (2002) A review of the assessment and treatment of anger and aggression in offenders with intellectual disability. *Journal of Intellectual Disability Research*, **46**, 57–73.
15. Dagnan, D., Chadwick, P. and Proudlove, J. (2000) Toward assessment of suitability of people with mental retardation for cognitive therapy. *Cognitive Therapy and Research*, **24**, 627–636.
16. Joyce, T., Globe, A. and Moody, C. (2006) Assessment of the component skills for cognitive therapy in adults with intellectual disabilities. *Journal of Applied Research in Intellectual Disabilities*, **19**, 17–23.
17. Symington, N. (1981) The psychotherapy of a subnormal patient. *British Journal of Medical Psychology*, **54**, 187–199.
18. Frankish, P. (1992) A psychodynamic approach to emotional difficulties within a social framework. *Journal of Intellectual Disability Research*, **36**, 295–305.
19. Hollins, S. and Sinason, V. (2000) Psychotherapy, learning disabilities and trauma: new perspectives. *British Journal of Psychiatry*, **176**, 37–41.
20. Hodges, S. (2003) *Counselling Adults with Learning Disabilities*, Palgrave Macmillan, Basingstoke.
21. Beail, N. (1995) Evaluation of a psychodynamic psychotherapy service for adults with intellectual disabilities: rationale, design and preliminary outcome data. *Journal of Applied Research in Intellectual Disabilities*, **9**, 223–228.
22. Beail, N., Warden, S., Morsley, K. and Newman, D. (2005) Naturalistic evaluation of the effectiveness of psychodynamic psychotherapy with adults with intellectual disabilities. *Journal of Applied Research in Intellectual Disabilities*, **18**, 245–251.
23. Newman, D.W. and Beail, N. (2002) Monitoring change in psychotherapy with people with intellectual disabilities: the application of the assimilation of problematic experiences scale. *Journal of Applied Research in Intellectual Disabilities*, **15**, 48–60.
24. Seligman, M. and Darling, R.B. (2007) *Ordinary Families, Special Children: A Systems Approach to Childhood Disability*, 33rd edn, Guilford, New York.
25. Baum S. and Lynggaard H. (eds) (2006) *Intellectual Disabilities: A Systemic Approach*, Karnac, London.
26. Fredman G. (2006) Working systemically with intellectual disability: why not? in *Intellectual Disabilities: A Systemic Approach* (eds S. Baum and H. Lynggaard), Karnac, London, pp. 1–20.
27. Vetere A. (1993) Using family therapy in services for people with learning disabilities, in *Using Family Therapy in the 90s* (eds J. Carpenter and A. Treacher), Blackwell, Oxford.
28. Goldberg, D., Magrill, L., Hale, J. *et al.* (1995) Protection and loss: working with learning disabled adults and their families. *Journal of Family Therapy*, **17**, 263–280.
29. Department of Health (2001) *Valuing People: A New Strategy for Learning Disability for the 21st Century*, HMSO, London.
30. Lynggaard H. and Baum S. (2006) So how do I . . . ? in *Intellectual Disabilities: A Systemic Approach* (eds S. Baum and H. Lynggaard), Karnac, London, pp. 185–202.
31. Oliver, P.C., Piachaud, J., Done, J. *et al.* (2002) Difficulties in conducting a randomised controlled trial of health service interventions in intellectual disability: implications for evidence based practice. *Journal of Intellectual disability Research*, **46**, 340–345.

32. Taylor, J.L., Novaco, R.W., Gillmer, B.T. *et al.* (2005) Individual cognitive-behavioural anger treatment for people with mild-borderline intellectual disabilities and histories of aggression: a controlled trial. *British Journal of Clinical Psychology*, **44**, 367–382.

33. Mason, J. (2007) The provision of psychological therapy to people with intellectual disabilities: an investigation into some of the relevant factors. *Journal of Intellectual Disability Research*, **51**, 244–249.

Further reading

Journal of Applied Research in Intellectual Disabilities, (2006) Special issue on cognitive behaviour therapy, **19** (1).

16 Community Care

Philip Dodd[1] and Patricia Noonan Walsh[2]

[1]St Michael's House, Dublin, Ireland
[2]Centre for Disability Studies, University College Dublin, Ireland

16.1 The development of care – an historical perspective

Early history

Attitudes and care perspectives to people with disabilities can be traced back to ancient Greece, where the omnipotent ideal body shape and fitness were linked to the accepted practice of infanticide for those children born with visible impairments. Indeed the Bible contains examples of cases where an individual's physical or mental impairments were seen as a punishment for past sins. More positively, one of the first hospitals described was founded in 1284 AD by the Sultan of Egypt, which contained a department of psychiatry, providing care to people with intellectual disabilities among other patient groups.

In general in pre-industrial (feudal) times, people with severe disabilities had very poor survival rates. However, less disabled individuals were expected to work in agriculture, if able, or resort to begging to supplement the family income. This may have contributed to an overall acceptance of people with disabilities in general in society, without the need for segregation; [1] care, though very basic, was within the family and the community. With the industrial revolution came a qualitative shift in attitudes to disabilities, placing the disability as very much a personal tragedy, with reduced tolerance at family and community levels [2].

Colonial expansion in the sixteenth century brought in its wake a model of care in special institutions. The first mental hospital in the Americas, San Hipólito, was established in Mexico City in 1566 through the efforts of a Spanish philanthropist [3].

Intellectual Disability Psychiatry: a practical handbook   Angela Hassiotis, Diana Andrea Barron and Ian Hall (eds)
© 2009 John Wiley & Sons, Ltd

Nineteenth century onwards

The development of specific care to people with intellectual disabilities, as opposed to those with mental illness or epilepsy, is hard to sketch historically. The work of French physician Jean-Marc Itard is often quoted as the first description of a care approach to an individual with apparent intellectual disabilities, which was developed upon by Seguin, developing specific services in France and the USA which were education-based and in a spirit of therapeutic optimism (see Case vignette 16.1).

Case vignette 16.1   Victor, the 'Wild Boy of Aveyron'

Victor was first sighted wandering in the woods near Saint Sernin sur Rance, in southern France, in 1797. He was captured at the age of 12, having previously been abandoned by his family. He was unable to speak and had a number of scars on his body, suggesting that he had been in the wild for some time.

Victor was taken to the National Institute for the Deaf in Paris, where he met physician Itard, who proposed to try and teach the young boy some speech and language skills, as well as 'civilized' behaviour, including empathy.

Itard's partial success in helping Victor was well publicized and his case became the focus of many to advance the principals described by the philosophy of the 'Enlightenment' in Western countries. Itard's ideas around the provision of education and training to people that were previously considered unsuitable, such as Victor, were considered to be revolutionary and visionary.

Victor is considered by many to be the first documented case of autism. He died at the age of 40 in Paris.

However, by the mid nineteenth century, many people with intellectual disabilities, along with people with mental illness and neurological diseases, were housed in a wide ranging institutional system, including hospitals, asylums, prisons, workhouses, industrial schools and colonies [4].

Gradually, the distinctive characteristics of persons with intellectual disabilities were recognized, leading to separate provision. In Ireland, Stewart's Hospital opened in west County Dublin in 1869, benefiting from a successful appeal for philanthropic funds. Dr Henry Hutchinson Stewart offered to provide not only care, but also education, for child residents with intellectual disabilities, or *idiot children*, who were called pupils rather than patients [5].

With continued industrialization came a change of emphasis in priorities of care. Early institutions were often small, and had rudimentary aims of rehabilitation, treatment and discharge. However, as the state started to become more involved in care provision, institutions grew exponentially in size, with long-term incarceration the result. In the United States, one response to overcrowding in mental institutions at the end of the nineteenth century was the gradual development of family care for people with mental illness through placing them in the homes of unrelated families. This model of care had its inception in Massachusetts, and represented the first efforts to provide state-sponsored services in community settings: however, family care never became widespread in the United States [3].

Eugenics

As the evolutionary ideas of Charles Darwin spread in the early twentieth century, impairment and disability became seen as a threat to social progress. The eugenic theory was developed by statisticians initially in the nineteenth century, but then inaccurately generalized by many parts of society. The eugenic theory indicated that the disproportionate growth of 'moral imbeciles' (which included people with intellectual disabilities) threatened the very survival of the 'race', as described by Darwin. Eugenicists highlighted apparent links between intellectual (and physical) disabilities, and other social ills such as alcoholism, crime, prostitution, unemployment and homelessness. Throughout North America and Europe, policies promoting 'social hygiene' developed, ranging from segregation in institutions, to state sponsored schemes of sterilization and abortion.

In Germany, Karl Binding, a legal scholar, argued that the lives of those suffering from 'incurable feeblemindedness' were purposeless. These individuals were described as being *lebensunwert*, or *unworthy of life*, yet their care absorbed immense resources from society [6]. Binding and Alfred Hoche, a scholarly psychiatrist, developed many of the arguments that were adopted by the Nazi killers in promoting euthanasia, and subsequently in carrying out the systematic extermination of hundreds of thousands of children.

The total institution

Eugenic ideas had a huge influence on the conditions that people with intellectual disabilities had to live with in the very large institutions that developed. In relative contrast to people with primary mental illness or neurological disease, there was limited interest in researching the needs of people with intellectual disabilities or improving their education, rehabilitation or care.

From the 1950s onwards, segregated institutions attracted growing criticism, both from people with disabilities, patients, as well as social reformers and politicians. Goffman [7] described the psychiatric asylum as the 'total institution', where the institution, rather than the 'patients' was the priority. An inmate's privacy, individuality, respect, protection and dignity were routinely ignored.

Deinstitutionalization

Institutional census figures swelled into the mid twentieth century, reaching a high water mark in the United States as late as 1967 [8]. Many thousands of people with intellectual disabilities lived quite separate, and certainly unequal, lives throughout these and other developed countries. Social invisibility brought its own risks: notoriously, residents of the Willowbrook institution on Staten Island in New York – at one time housing more than 4000 individuals – were exposed to hepatitis B for experimental purposes without their knowledge or consent [3].

What fuelled the dramatic, if incomplete, reversal away from huge institutions towards small-scale, community care? The springs of this sea change flowed in part from radical thinking about the injustice of segregation and the primacy of self-determination and normalization. The principle of normalization had developed since the mid twentieth century in the Nordic countries, and a key contributor, Niels Erik Bank-Mikkelsen in Denmark, set its goal as normalizing – not individuals, but rather – the living conditions of people with disabilities. This might be achieved through creating situations for people with disabilities that were as near normal as possible [9]. Arguably, three main forces helped to drive deinstitutionalization in the United States: the voices of families and other concerned citizens seeking alternatives; a new interest in normalization; and growing awareness of often horrific conditions in large institutions [8]. In England, scandals about large residential hospitals in the 1960s reached the public and provoked scrutiny.

The process of deinstitutionalization of citizens with intellectual disabilities in the past 40 years has varied in pace. It has concluded in some parts of the world – in Sweden, for example [10]. In other countries it is still an aspiration, or perhaps a goal not yet visualized for people with intellectual disabilities. Many countries have undergone fits and starts in the journey towards community living, due to lack of leadership, the strength of forces that maintain a dual-track system of care, and many other complex political and social factors that serve to retain vast institutions focused on segregated care.

In the main, evidence about the impact of deinstitutionalization, a particular social policy, rests on studies undertaken in the UK and USA after the purposeful closure of large state-operated facilities that were widely acknowledged to be in a state of crisis [11]. The journey towards community living was not even, and it is evident that the pace of and response to deinstitutionalization varied markedly. For example, transformation in Michigan in the United States was swift:

> During the 1970s and 1980s, the convergence of leadership by advocates, legislators, and bureaucrats led to Michigan's rapid transformation from an institutional to a community-based system, which was further facilitated by a political culture open to innovation [8; p. 219].

By contrast, a lack of leadership, augmented by politically powerful groups of the parents of institutionalized persons and large providers, in nearby Illinois resulted in a slower rate of change and a dual system of provision – both community and institutional services – that persists.

In Australia, large-scale deinstitutionalization took place some 20 years after similar movements in North America and Europe. However, individuals with intellectual disabilities living in Australian institutions moved directly into small group community homes for five or fewer residents, rather than larger or intermediate purpose-built residences as was the case in the United States and the UK [12].

In Sweden, various Acts of Parliament since the mid twentieth century had gradually led to the closure of institutions and the development of community-based services: an Act in 1985 'for the first time, clarified the right for everyone with an intellectual disability, even those with a severe form, to participate in community life' [13].

Case vignette 16.2

In Sweden today, Maria, a young woman with severe intellectual disabilities, lives contentedly in her own home, one of two adjoined homes on a leafy street in a small town. Her house is not remarkable in any way. There are neighbours close at hand, and a homely living room decorated by Maria's mother is the place to entertain guests and hold parties. She visits her family each month and for some holidays – other holidays are spent travelling in Europe. An array of supports are in place so that Maria can live an active life with full-time assistance and companionship from support workers whom she helps her parents to recruit directly, but whose salary is paid by the local municipality.

16.2 Modern mental health services for people with intellectual disabilities

The rights of people with intellectual disabilities to access mainstream generic as well as specialist mental health services has been national policy in a number of jurisdictions [14, 15]. However, in many countries, no specific policies are in place outlining mental health care for this population.

History and local service legacies have been shown to have a huge influence on the pattern of development of mental health services for people with intellectual disabilities. As a result, a whole range of approaches to service provision exists, which at best encourages innovation and high quality services but, at worst, presents as exclusionary, with unclear care pathways [16]. There exists a huge diversity in levels of expertise, staffing levels and funding options. Service use and need vary according to local circumstances and demographic profiles.

General service delivery

Agreement around the best structure and system of providing mental health services to people with intellectual disabilities is less than clear.

In a number of countries, and especially in the UK, the community intellectual disability team developed to provide general supports to people with intellectual disabilities in the community. Though psychiatrists often worked as part of these teams, most of the work of the teams initially maintained a general, non-specialist focus. Later they have developed some specialization, such as specialist mental health care (see Box 16.1).

Box 16.1   The community intellectual disability team

Services provided

- Assessment of intellectual disabilities and associated health and social care needs

- Care packages to address social care needs including

    - day service opportunities

    - employment

    - support to manage tenancy

    - personal care

- Support to access mainstream primary and secondary healthcare services

- Specialist health care interventions, including

    - mental health and challenging behaviour

    - communication

    - physiotherapy

    - aids and adaptions to the environment

- Training local service providers

- Supporting local service developments.

Professions involved
- Speech and language therapy

- Physiotherapy

- Nursing

- Social work

- Occupational therapy

- Psychiatry

- Psychology

- Psychotherapy.

Case vignette 16.3

Jean is a 41-year-old woman with a mild intellectual disability. Since her mother died seven years ago, she has been living in a residential home with people with more severe disabilities than herself. She has always wanted to live independently. She has a history of hypothyroidism and inflammatory bowel disease, as well as a past history of moderate depressive illness, that required a brief hospital admission. She is taking a number of medicines, but her health is overall very stable. A year ago, the local community intellectual disability team began to support her to explore the possibilities of living independently.

The team psychologist assessed Jean's adaptive skills, and set up a trial placement in an independent residential unit, with significant staff inputs to assess Jean's abilities to live independently. The social worker supported Jean and her family as they resolved anxieties or worries that they may have had with the move, as well as maximizing entitled welfare benefits. The team psychiatrist, psychologist, general practitioner and nurse, as well as Jean and her family put together a health plan, along with specific training to care staff regarding Jean's health needs, to ensure that all involved with Jean were aware of the specific risks and care priorities, to best protect Jean from a relapse in her various medical and mental health conditions.

Jean moved into her own apartment three months ago. A care worker calls to her every day, and she uses a specifically designed electronic communication system to contact care staff should she need it. Her care manager is now helping Jean to find a job close to her new apartment.

Learning points

- Case vignette 16.3 illustrates a person centred approach to care provision, whereby the wishes of the client are the basis of the service.

- Despite the fact that a number of obstacles existed for the client to achieve true community living, the various members of the community intellectual disability team worked to overcome these obstacles.

- Community orientated care provision is resource intensive.

- The success of this case is based on ongoing support and evaluation.

European models

In general, with deinstitutionalization, there has been a growing reliance on families, voluntary and private agencies to provide long-term care. European countries have tended to develop mental health and intellectual disability policies and services separately, with many problematic gaps in care. Few models have been reported; one study looked at the range of service models in five European countries including Austria, Greece, England, Ireland and Spain [17]. This study found that, for the most part, policy and legislation in the countries that were studied tended to separate the disability aspects of people with intellectual disabilities from their mental health needs, with the result that the service needs of this population were largely going unnoticed.

Some intensive community treatment models have been assessed: a Dutch-based randomized control trial showed reduced levels of hospitalization from assertive services based within intellectual disability community services [18].

USA

In general, there are few evaluated services reported from the USA. Complex health insurance arrangements, as well as differing state policies, make for a lack of consensus in service delivery. A model developed in New York has shown that a comprehensive service can be developed when existing services come together to try to design a cohesive service, and define clear care pathways [19]. A second service in the New York area has also been evaluated, which consisted of a range of intellectual disability services, with access to a comprehensive mental health service, the success of both services being dependent on each other [20].

Canada

A process of rapid deinstitutionalization led to the development of many small mental health centres of care. A lack of trained psychiatrists has delayed the development of larger-scale services. A specialist service in Toronto developed from a number of generic intellectual disability agencies coming together to develop shared mental health services. Assessment and treatment planning is the focus of care, with a crisis intervention team in place to try to support community treatment as much as possible, to avoid hospital admission [21].

Australia

A novel approach to the management of challenging behaviour was developed in Queensland, starting with an extensive assessment of the incidence, prevalence and risk factors associated with the behaviour. A successful 'train-the trainers' approach was developed [22] in the delivery of training of behavioural support. A carer consultation, training and education programme has been developed in Melbourne, [23] which has influenced state mental health policy development.

Patterns of service development

In many countries, including the UK, government policy suggests that mental health services for people with intellectual disabilities should develop from mainstream mental health services. Indeed this type of service provision is in keeping with concepts associated with normalization. However, in practice, mainstream community mental health teams have found it increasingly difficult to meet the needs of people with intellectual disabilities with complex mental health problems [24]. Box 16.2 outlines the components of an ideal mental health service for people with intellectual disabilities.

Box 16.2   Components of an ideal mental health service for people with intellectual disabilities

- Coordinated, comprehensive and culturally competent delivery of service

- Full access to assessment, treatment and support services

- Continuity of care

- Therapeutic interventions supported by evidence-based practices

- Pharmacological treatment based on efficacy

- Support services for housing, employment and leisure activities

- Assist in improving independence and quality of life.

In practice, mental health services have developed from within the social services and primary care led intellectual disability services, through the partial specialization of the community intellectual disability team referred to above.

There are challenges to this type of approach: there needs to be a range of mental health professionals within the community team, not just a lone psychiatrist. It is important not to duplicate services provided elsewhere: for example crisis intervention teams that provide a 24-hour service, and psychiatric admission facilities for people with acute relapses of mental illness (see Chapter 13 for a discussion of the management of mental health crises). However, people with intellectual disabilities can find mainstream inpatient services problematic [25]. There can be boundary disputes between intellectual disability services and mainstream mental health services regarding clinical and service responsibility, making care pathways difficult. These problems can, however, be largely prevented by agreeing local protocols between mainstream mental health services and intellectual disability services [26].

Some success has been shown with this type of service: a Dutch-based randomized control trial showed reduced levels of hospitalization from services based within intellectual disability services [18]. Bouras and colleagues have developed and evaluated extensively a mental health service in London, which is delivered from generic mental health services, but has outreach consultation and training in community intellectual disability service providers. This has the benefit of having clear access to both secondary and tertiary level specialized acute treatment when needed, but much of the outpatient support services provided by the community intellectual disability services [24]. Individuals admitted to the tertiary level treatment unit showed a significant decrease in psychiatric symptoms, an increase in overall level of functioning and an improvement in behavioural problems on discharge, compared to a similar sample treated in the generic treatment unit, at six and twelve months post discharge [27]. Good outcomes have also been reported for a more integrated model with mental health and intellectual disability services providing a joint service in an inpatient setting and through a community 'virtual team' [28].

Specific approaches to care in the UK

The care programme approach (CPA) [29] is a system of care delivered to individuals within specialist mental services, whereby their health and social care needs are assessed, care plans are formulated, all coordinated by a key worker, in a systematic, homogenous system. Much debate has centred around the threshold of mental health need, that indicates when an individual should benefit from CPA. This is especially pertinent when one considers people presenting primarily with behavioural problems, without a clear psychiatric diagnosis [30]. Applying the CPA to people with intellectual disabilities and mental health problems should lead to greater joint working between intellectual disability and generic mental health services.

Assertive community treatment (ACT)

Assertive community treatment (ACT) is a service model developed in the USA for those individuals with severe and persistent psychiatric illness, with little community support; relevant cases usually experienced frequent relapse, with associated readmission to hospital. Assertive outreach (previously referred to as intensive case management) is widely assumed to contain many of the components of the original ACT model.

In a study of intensive case management (the UK 700 study), people with borderline or mild intellectual disabilities spent less time in hospital if they receive intensive rather than standard community care [31].

Problems exist as to what constitutes ACT or assertive outreach in intellectual disability mental health services, as a number of different configurations exist, despite many of them being described as assertive outreach. This makes for difficulties in comparing like services with like for the purposes of evaluating efficacy.

Supporting care staff

As care has shifted from a predominantly institutional care setting to community-based services, family members and paid carers have moved to the centre stage of care provision for this population. Paid staff represents a significant part of the workforce. In many parts of the world, large proportions of staff are unqualified, are on low pay and are predominantly young, and often inexperienced. They may find themselves working with individuals with significant mental health or behavioural problems, sometimes without having acquired the skills to do so, and without expert professional support.

Staff working in intellectual disability services experienced more psychological distress compared with general workers, or staff working in the health services in general [32]. However, when work distress is more clearly defined, it would appear that staff working with people with intellectual disabilities in general have a lower level of occupational 'burnout' (Box 16.3), when compared to staff working in other human services [33]. The underlying cause of this is unclear, although may relate to the many positive and rewarding aspects of working with people with intellectual disabilities.

Box 16.3   Burnout

'Burnout' is defined as the emotional and mental exhaustion, loss of feelings of accomplishment, as well as depersonalized attitudes towards service users.
   Factors associated with front-line staff work stress and burnout:

• Poor support from colleagues, managers, supervisors

• Staff feeling unclear about their role, and feeling conflicted in work demands

• Poor working conditions

• Unqualified staff, with a sense of wanting more training

• Staff having a negative perception of the job and a lack of commitment.

An important contribution that psychiatrists can make to reduce staff stress is to contribute to front line staff training for staff supporting people with mental health problems. This is a core role for community intellectual disability teams. A number of excellent training resources are available to assist in this [34].

Case vignette 16.4

For many years, Sarah had worked part-time in the kitchen of the head office of a human services organization located in an industrial park. A professional worker dropped in regularly to ensure that both Sarah and the host company were content with her employment. She was deft in all the tasks assigned to her: preparing sandwiches, soup and tea, wiping down work surfaces, setting trays for meetings and loading the dishwasher. She signed for her weekly pay packet and always planned her budget. Since her youth – when she had attended a nearby sheltered workshop as a trainee – Sarah had taken pride in what she did and also in her well-groomed appearance. She responded warmly to the attention of the staff and greeted each visitor with courtesy.

During the winter months around the time of her forty-fifth birthday, some incidents provoked concern. Often, Sarah seemed to ignore greetings and requests, keeping her back turned even from the staff members she had known for a long time. Although she completed daily tasks, her manner was distant, and when finally she might turn her attention to a request, she shouted her reply. Some mornings, Sarah appeared unkempt and became irritable when prompted to change her apron or wash her hands. Reluctantly the management decided that as Sarah's behaviour had become troublesome, she was no longer valuable in her current role. Plans were afoot to guide her in transferring to another form of day activity with support.

Just before her transfer, Sarah's professional support worker consulted a newly appointed registrar in psychiatry who asked, first, whether Sarah had recently had a health check; they found that she had not, and the community nurse supported Sarah to have the check. The results of screening indicated that Sarah's hearing was substantially impaired in both ears; she simply could not hear the questions and requests of her colleagues, nor did she understand what had been happening, and thus avoided speaking with others or shouted at them. She had become so anxious that her well-honed practices of good grooming and personal shopping had faded. Sarah adjusted well to hearing aids and, once guided about her changed hearing status, she continued to work.

The psychiatric registrar, Dr Murphy, spoke with her health colleagues and other staff members, finding strong interest in learning more about health of the persons whom they supported. She set up brief training sessions together with the community nurse that became part of the induction and continuous training programme for care staff.

Learning points

- People with intellectual disability are likely to incur secondary mental and physical health conditions throughout their lives, some of which may be manifested in behaviours that are perceived as challenging.

- Hearing and visual impairments are prevalent among adults with intellectual disabilities.

- As community-based arrangements for living and working increase, a more diverse group of individuals will be in contact with persons with intellectual disability, and may not understand their health needs.

- Community intellectual disabilities teams have an important role in both identifying health needs and training other staff to do so.

16.3 Conclusion

Cultural and political attitudes towards people with intellectual disabilities have changed through many ages since Greek and Roman times, up to the present day. Mirroring this, care provision has varied significantly from complete institutional state care to unsupported family centred care.

Modern Western care provision is now primarily community-based. Historic care legacies continue to influence the development of modern services. Modern mental health services for people with intellectual disabilities have either developed as part of general intellectual disability services (e.g. the community intellectual disability team), or else have developed into specialist service teams focussed primarily on mental health care. Evidence exists that indicates that both of these approaches to mental health care are effective.

References

1. Oliver, M. and Barnes, C. (1998) *Social Policy and Disabled People: From Exclusion to Inclusion*, Longman, London.
2. Finkelstein V. (1983) Disability and the helper/helped relationship: an historical view, in *Handicap in a Social World* (eds A. Brechin P. Liddiard and J. Swaine), Hodder & Stoughton, Milton Keynes.
3. Braddock D. and Parish S. (2001) An institutional history of disability, in *Handbook of Disability Studies* (eds G. Albrecht, K.D. Seelman and M. Bury), Sage Publications, Thousand Oaks, pp. 11–68.

4. Cohen, S. and Scull, A. (1983) *Social Control and the State*, Blackwell, Oxford.

5. Robins, J. (1986) *Fools and Mad: A History of the Insane in Ireland*, Institute of Public Administration, Dublin.

6. Friedlander, H. (1995) *The Origins of Nazi Genocide*, University of North Carolina Press, Chapel Hill and London.

7. Goffman, E. (1961) *Asylums: Essays on the Social Situation of Mental Patients and Other Inmates*, Doubleday, New York.

8. Parish, S. (2005) Deinstitutionalization in two states: the impact of advocacy, policy, and other social forces on services for people with developmental disabilities. *Research and Practice for Persons with Severe Disabilities*, **30**, 219–231.

9. Parmenter, T. (2006) Normalization, in *Encyclopaedia of Disability*, Vol. 3 (eds G.L. Albrecht J. Bickenbach D.T. Mitchell *et al.*), Sage Publications, Thousand Oaks, pp 1157–1160.

10. Beadle-Brown, J., Mansell, J. and Kozma, A. (2007) Deinstitutionalization in intellectual disabilities. *Current Opinion in Psychiatry*, **20**, 437–442.

11. Emerson, E., McConkey, R., Walsh, P. and Felce, D. (2008) Intellectual disability in a global context. *Journal of Policy and Practice in Intellectual Disability*, **5** (2), 79–80.

12. Young, L. and Ashman, A. (2004) Deinstitutionalization in Australia part I: historical perspective. *British Journal of Developmental Disabilities*, **50**, 21–28.

13. Ericsson, K. (2000) Deinstitutionalization and community living for persons with an intellectual disability in Sweden: policy, organizational change and personal consequences. Presentation, Disability Conference, Tokyo [cited February 2009]. Available from: http://www.skinfaxe.se/ebok/tokyo.pdf.

14. Department of Health (2001) *Valuing People: A New Strategy for Learning Disabilities in the 21st Century*, HMSO, London.

15. Department of Health and Children (2006) *A Vision for Change: Report of the Expert Group on Mental Health Policy*, The Stationary Office, Dublin.

16. Hassiotis, A., Barron, P. and O'Hara, J. (2000) Mental health services for people with learning disabilities. *British Medical Journal*, **321**, 583–584.

17. Holt, G., Costello, H., Bouras, N. *et al.* (2000) BIOMED-MEROPE project: service provision for adults with intellectual disabilities: a European comparison. *Journal of Intellectual Disability Research*, **44** (6), 685–696.

18. Van Minnen, A., Hoogduin, C.A.L. and Broekman, T.G. (1997) Hospital vs. outreach treatment of patients with mental retardation and psychiatric disorders: a controlled study. *Acta Psychiatrica Scandinavica*, **95**, 515–522.

19. Davidson, P.W., Cain, N. and Sloane-Reeves, J. (1995) Crisis intervention for community based individuals with developmental disabilities and behavioural and psychiatric disorders. *Mental Retardation*, **33**, 21–30.

20. Landsberg, G., Fletcher, F. and Maxwell, T. (1987) Developing a comprehensive community care system for the mentally ill/mentally retarded. *Community Mental Health Journal*, **23**, 137–142.

21. Pudddephatt, A. and Sussman, S. (1994) Developing services in Canada: Ontario vignettes, in *Mental Health in Mental Retardation: Recent Advances and Practices* (ed. N. Bouras), Cambridge University Press, Cambridge.

22. Attwood T. and Joachin R. (1994) The prevention and management of seriously disruptive behaviour in Australia, in *Mental Health in Mental Retardation: Recent Advances and Practices* (ed. N. Bouras), Cambridge University Press, Cambridge.

23. Bennet, C. (2000) The Victorian dual disability service. *Australasian Psychiatry*, **8** (3), 238–243.

24. Bouras, N. and Holt, G. (2001) Community mental health service for adults with learning disabilities, in *Textbook of Community Psychiatry* (eds G. Thornicroft and G. Smukler), Oxford University Press, Oxford, pp. 97–407.

25. Parkes, C., Samuels, S., Hassiotis, A. *et al.* (2007) Incorporating the views of service users in the development of an integrated psychiatric service for people with learning disabilities. *British Journal of Learning Disabilities*, **35**, 23–29.

26. Foundation for People with Learning Disabilities (2004) Green Light for Mental Health, Foundation for People with Learning Disabilities, London.

27. Xenitidis, K., Gratsa, A., Bouras, N. *et al.* (2004) Psychiatric inpatient cares for adults with intellectual disabilities: generic or specialist units? *Journal of Intellectual Disability Research*, **48**, 11–18.

28. Hall, I., Parkes, C., Samuels, S. and Hassiotis, A. (2006) Working across boundaries: clinical outcomes for an integrated mental health service for people with intellectual disabilities. *Journal of Intellectual Disability Research*, **50**, 598–607.

29. Department of Health (1999) Effective Care Co-ordination in Mental Health Services: Modernizing the CPA, Department of Health, London.

30. Roy, A. (2000) The care programme approach in learning disability psychiatry. *Advances in Psychiatric Treatment*, **6**, 380–387.

31. Hassiotis, A., Ukoumunne, O. and Byford, S. (2001) Intellectual functioning and outcome of patients with severe psychotic illness randomised to intensive case management: report from the UK700 trial. *British Journal of Psychiatry*, **178**, 166–171.

32. Hatton, C., Emerson, E. and Rivers, M. (1999) Factors associated with staff stress and work satisfaction in services for people with intellectual disabilities. *Journal of Intellectual Disabilities Research*, **43**, 253–270.

33. Skirrow, P. and Hatton, P. (2007) 'Burnout' amongst direct care workers in services for adults with intellectual disabilities: a systematic review of research findings and initial normative data. *Journal of Applied Research in Intellectual Disabilities*, **20**, 131–144.

34. Holt, G., Hardy, S. and Bouras, N. (2005) *Mental Health in Learning Disabilities: A Training Resource*, Pavilion, London.

Appendix A

Critique of the ICD 10 and DSM IV based Classification of Mental Disorders in Intellectual Disability

Anna Cooper[1] and Angela Hassiotis[2]

[1]Division of Community Based Sciences, University of Glasgow, UK
[2]Department of Mental Health Services, University College London, UK

The introduction of the *ICD-10 Clinical Descriptions and Diagnostic Guidelines* and *ICD-10 Diagnostic Criteria for Research* provided a major step forward in world psychiatric research and practice. However, for adults with intellectual disabilities, this classificatory system, and the criteria within several of the disorders, are difficult to apply. Consequently, despite the much higher prevalence of psychiatric disorders in this population compared with the general population, [1] the anticipated advances in diagnostic practice and in psychiatric research have not taken place. Most published studies on adults with intellectual disabilities have modified the criteria offered by the existing classification systems in order to increase their utility. Such modifications are not always cited in full, differ between studies and render comparisons of findings or synthesis of evidence difficult [2–4].

The Royal College of Psychiatrists, UK, attempted to address the problem with the publication of DC-LD in 2001, [5] which was designed to complement ICD-10, and the National Association for the Dually Diagnosed in association with the American Psychiatric Association published DM-ID [6] in 2008, due to similar problems with DSM-IV-TR. Previously, WHO raised awareness of the

Intellectual Disability Psychiatry: a practical handbook   Angela Hassiotis, Diana Andrea Barron and Ian Hall (eds)
© 2009 John Wiley & Sons, Ltd

diagnostic difficulties and differences presented by adults with intellectual disabilities when attempting to apply ICD-10 criteria by publishing the *ICD-10 Guide for Mental Retardation* [7]. This demonstrates that WHO established the principle that the standard ICD-10 does not, on its own, fully address the psychiatric disorders experienced by adults with intellectual disabilities.

In a clinical context, staff working in mainstream psychiatric services spend most of their time looking after the general population, and are unlikely to be aware of the pathoplastic effect of severity of intellectual deficit on psychopathology. An accurate description of the psychiatric disorders that adults and older people experience and its presentation is important so that staff have a guide to help them to recognize such disorders, and therefore initiate appropriate treatment.

Below we set examples of problems seen in the utility of ICD-10 for adults with intellectual disabilities:

1. *Problem behaviours* are the most common type of psychiatric disorders experienced by adults with intellectual disabilities. They are remitting-relapsing disorders, with incident episodes related to biological, psychological, social and developmental aetiologies. Within the ICD-10 the F70-79 codes are used to define such behaviours under the terms 'no, or minimal, impairment of behaviour', 'significant impairment of behaviour requiring attention or treatment', 'other impairments of behaviour' or 'without mention of impairment of behaviour'. Within *ICD-10 Clinical Descriptions and Diagnostic Guidelines*, and *ICD-10 Diagnostic Criteria for Research*, the specifier does not clarify whether the type of behaviour being referred to is adaptive behaviour or problem behaviour. It does not distinguish between problem behaviours occurring as a psychiatric disorder, or occurring merely as a symptom of some other disorder (primary or secondary problem behaviours), for example a symptom of depression, or a symptom of tooth ache; this is important as the correct diagnosis is a guide towards the most appropriate interventions. Additionally, the specifier does not include operationalized criteria, and so is likely to lead to different usage by different clinicians/researchers. The *ICD-10 Guide for Mental Retardation* refers to problem behaviour and abnormal behaviour and adds a further specifier for some types of problem behaviour, but does not operationalize these.

2. *Clinical presentations* of some disorders differ from those found within the general population with increasing levels of intellectual disabilities. For example, the main mood symptom found in depressive episodes is often irritability rather than misery. Depressive episodes also often present with loss of adaptive behaviour skills, reduced communication, social withdrawal, onset of or increase in problem behaviours and reassurance-seeking behaviour, which are not listed as criteria in ICD-10 depressive episodes (F32), together with sleep and appetite disturbance [8].

3. *Complex and sophisticated criteria* within ICD-10 are unlikely to be met by adults with intellectual disabilities even though they have the psychiatric disorder in question. A developmental age of about seven years has to be reached in order to comprehend the concepts of guilt and death. This will never be achieved by an adult with severe or profound intellectual disabilities as, by definition, it has an upper limit of mental age equivalent to six years. *Specific phobias* (F40.2) require the person to recognize that the fear they experience is disproportionate to the stimulus. Such information cannot be elicited from persons with severe or profound intellectual disabilities; however, their fear can be observed to be disproportionate to the stimulus. Rituals within *obsessive-compulsive disorder* (F42) can be observed, but the person may not be able to self-report that they are excessive or unreasonable, or that he/she tries to resist them.

4. Some *genetic causes* of intellectual disabilities have an associated behavioural phenotype that includes psychiatric disorders, such as dementia in Down's syndrome; self-injurious behaviour in Smith-Magenis syndrome; affective psychosis in Prader-Willi syndrome; psychosis in velo-cardio facial syndrome. The published literature on these disorders is unclear, due to lack of instruction in ICD-10 as to where these disorders should be coded. Some researchers have classified these as additional psychiatric disorders; some have included them in the organic categories (even though the criteria that the condition recovers when the underlying organic condition abates cannot be met, as the syndrome is lifelong). Others do not classify the psychiatric disorder at all, considering it a part of the genetic syndrome that causes intellectual disabilities. These latter two approaches may generate therapeutic nihilism, whereas some of these disorders can be ameliorated by treatment.

5. The *organic codes* within the section on 'Personality and Behavioural Disorders and Other Mental Disorders due to Brain Disease, Damage and Dysfunction, F07' have resulted in conflicting and confused usage, with some published research applying the terms just because the adult has epilepsy (which is present in 25% of this population) in addition to the psychiatric disorder, or on the assumption that the intellectual disability is the cause of the psychiatric disorder. Such an approach is unhelpful in terms of guiding treatment choices or considering prognosis, and introduces problems in the interpretation of published literature.

6. A significant minority of adults with intellectual disabilities *lack a diagnostic assessments for ADHD or autism* in childhood due to services being underdeveloped. As adults they may clearly have all the symptoms of these conditions, sometimes to a severe extent, with the symptoms known to have been present for as long as any of their informants have known the person. However, in the absence of collateral information, a developmental history from early childhood can no longer be collected. If their medical notes do not include a contemporaneously recorded early developmental history (which is typically the case), the ICD-10

diagnosis of autism or ADHD cannot therefore be applied, as the age of onset cannot be determined.

These examples indicate that the classification of mental disorders in adults with intellectual disabilities should be addressed as a priority. In the light of the new revisions of the ICD and DSM now due, it is imperative that experts in all branches of psychiatry including expert panels in the psychiatry of intellectual disabilities, must work together to address the deficits of the existing diagnostic criteria. Such work has far reaching consequences for the quality of care of people with intellectual disabilities and the training and advances in research in this field.

References

1. Bailey, N.M. (2007) Prevalence of psychiatric disorders in adults with moderate to profound learning disabilities. *Advances in Mental Health and Learning Disabilities*, **2**, 36–44.
2. Sturmey, P. (1995) DSM-IIIR and persons with dual diagnoses: conceptual issues and strategies for future research. *Journal of Intellectual Disability Research*, **39**, 357–364.
3. Sturmey, P. (1995) Diagnostic-based pharmacological treatment of behaviour disorders in persons with developmental disabilities: a review and a decision-making typology. *Research on Developmental Disabilities*, **16**, 235–252.
4. Cooper, S-A., Melville, C.A., and Einfeld, S.L. (2003) Psychiatric diagnosis, intellectual disabilities and Diagnostic Criteria for Psychiatric Disorders for Use with Adults with Learning Disabilities/Mental retardation (DC-LD). *Journal of Intellectual Disability Research*, **47**, 3–15.
5. Royal College of Psychiatrists (2001) *DC-LD [Diagnostic Criteria for Psychiatric Disorders for Use with Adults with Learning Disabilities/Mental Retardation]*, Gaskell Press, London.
6. DM-ID A Clinical Guide for Diagnosis of Mental Disorders in Persons with Intellectual Disability, http://www.dmid.org/. Accessed in April 2009.
7. World Health Organization (1996) ICD-10 Guide for Mental Retardation, World Health Organization, Geneva.
8. Smiley, E. and Cooper, S.-A. (2003) Intellectual disabilities, depressive episode, diagnostic criteria and Diagnostic Criteria for Psychiatric Disorders for Use with Adults with Learning Disabilities/Mental retardation (DC-LD). *Journal of Intellectual Disability Research*, **47**, 62–71.

Appendix B

A to Z of Disciplines That May Contribute to the Multi- and Interdisciplinary Work as Applied to Mood and Anxiety Disorders*

Elspeth Bradley[1], Rebecca Goody[2] and Shirley McMillan[3]

[1]Department of Psychiatry, University of Toronto, Canada
[2]Cornwall Partnership NHS Trust, UK
[3]Surrey Place Centre, Toronto, Canada

This is not an exhaustive list but indicates some of the roles carried out by each discipline. The principles can also be applied to other mental disorders.

B.1 Audiology

• Hearing loss can present additional challenges to a person's communication and cognitive needs which in turn may to anxiety and mood disturbances.

• The audiologist can assess and prescribe interventions around the nature and extent of any hearing loss and refer onto other specialists.

* This list of professional framework is applicable to the management of other mental disorders in people with intellectual disabilities.

Intellectual Disability Psychiatry: a practical handbook   Angela Hassiotis, Diana Andrea Barron and Ian Hall (eds)
© 2009 John Wiley & Sons, Ltd

B.2 Behaviour therapy

Behaviour therapy (in some teams this work might be carried out by the behaviour specialist in conjunction with the nurse and/or psychologist) (also discussed in Chapter 15):

- A functional analysis of the person's behaviour may provide useful insight into a person's needs in relation to current and historical circumstances and identify environmental triggers and contingencies to mood and anxiety disturbances. The analysis does, however, require an interdisciplinary approach to incorporate wide ranging information into a coherent formulation [1, 2].

- The specialist may observe behaviours in the person's everyday environment not seen in the psychiatric interview, and as such may be able to provide details and a context to these behaviours so as to better understand their aetiology, for example panic attack as an explanation of 'aggression'.

- The specialist is able to operationalize behaviours that may be indicative of mood or anxiety disturbances. These can then be tracked systematically assisting diagnosis and monitoring of response to interventions (e.g. medication).

- Behavioural interventions can be targeted along a continuum of a person's escalating and maladaptive mood (and anxiety) arousal. Such interventions may include proactive/preventative strategies (e.g. teaching of new adaptive skills to person with intellectual disabilities, adapting social and physical environments to better support a person's needs) and/or reactive (e.g. medication as required, physical supports). However, where intrusive or restrictive strategies are required they must be within legal frameworks (e.g. criminal law, human rights, etc.) and regularly reviewed by the advising interdisciplinary team.

- The specialist can provide environmental assessments to ensure supports available to persons are appropriate to their needs and unique capacities (and not too stressful).

- The specialist can assist in implementing and auditing appropriate routine and medication administration practices.

- Work with care providers and interdisciplinary team members is key to effective and consistent behaviour therapy. This may include the provision of psycho-education to all relevant parties (including where possible people with intellectual disabilities, families and paid carers) about anxiety and mood.

There may also be the provision of advice about alternative, more adaptive, evidence-based approaches (e.g. assertiveness training for people experiencing anger, relaxation training for those experiencing stress) and how they might be adapted to better meet an individual's communication and cognitive styles and capacities.

B.3 Communication/speech-language pathology

- Assessment, treatment and prevention of language (expressive and receptive) and communication difficulties, particularly those contributing to the person's mood difficulties and anxiety levels, such as deficits with social communication and emotional expression.

- Direct interventions may include the development of person centred communication strategies and supports (e.g. use of visuals, social stories). Indirect interventions may include education to support networks about the person's communication needs and approaches to better meet those needs.

- Dysphagia and swallowing assessments.

B.4 Intake, service coordination and social work

Intake, service coordination and social work (referred to in a variety of ways including family support, case management, discharge planning in different agencies and in different health care settings). Services include:

- Meeting with families, other care providers and the individual to identify assessment, treatment and service needs and match those needs with the most appropriate services available within the team and/or in the local community.

- Assist in the development of a shared understanding of the situation to aid medical and psychosocial interventions.

- Link families, and/or individuals to recreational, respite, medical and financial resources in the community.

- Assist families in navigating the medical, social care and educational systems.

- Support persons living at home and their families. May include individual and family therapy.

B.5 Nursing

- Health assessments and referral to ensure that medical disorders contributing to anxiety or mood disturbances are identified.

- Work with family and hospital doctors and other community and hospital health providers to ensure health access and timely health care regardless of the patient's cognitive and communication impairments.

- Promote mental health and illnesses prevention. This includes group teaching such as women's health, men's health, healthy eating and exercise.

- Provide education and support individuals and their care providers, for example, as it relates to specific medication side effects.

B.6 Occupational therapy

- Person centred, collaboratively focussed assessment and intervention approaches acknowledging the dynamic relationship between persons, their environment and their occupations in order to assist them in being as functional and independent as they are able, including productivity (play, school and work), independent living (feeding, dressing, toileting, sleeping, basic hygiene issues) and leisure (recreational, social, play activities) skills; this may include assistive technology.

- Assessment and recommendations to support any sensory processing needs which contribute to a person's mood or anxiety state, especially individuals on the autism spectrum.

B.7 Other therapies

- Creative therapies such as art, music, drama, movement and dance. These are underpinned by psychological theories and psychotherapeutic approaches and can be provided to individuals and/or groups of people.

- Dietetics, particularly useful in relation to the high prevalence of obesity and behavioural difficulties around food and drinks, for example excessive consumption of substances, especially, but not limited to persons with Down and Prader-Willi syndromes.

- Counselling. As with the general population, many people with intellectual disabilities can benefit from various forms of counselling, as can the relatives coping with difficult situations.

B.8 Physiotherapy

- Assessment of psychomotor needs and development of therapeutic regimes, such as hydrotherapy.

- Functional assessments of gait and programmes to address concerns.

- Consultation around adaptations to assist in psychomotor activities, such as wheelchairs, walkers, canes and so on.

- Promotion of healthier lifestyles and physical education such as providing consultation around accessing and adapting mainstream exercise regimes.

B.9 Psychiatry

- Provides the medical and psychiatric perspective for persons referred for (i) assessment of concerns about anxiety, mood or other behavioural disturbances (ii) request for medication review (iii) request for second opinion.

- Provides psychiatric formulation and diagnosis.

- Supports and advocates for the interdisciplinary biopsychosocial work of the team. Ensure that non-medical interventions are fully supported (and resourced) and medical interventions offered only when this is good practice.

- Makes recommendations for further referrals for specialist medical and genetic consultation and assessments.

- May provide follow-up for outpatient and inpatient settings.

- Work together with other professionals, for example behaviour therapist monitoring target behaviours against medication response; psychologist in joint medication/psychotherapy treatment; occupational therapist in joint medication/ sensory treatment for clients with autism; speech language pathologist in assisting client communicate between emotional and physical distress

- Under the Mental Health Act can recommend compulsory treatment in hospital.

- Assesses the capacity of individuals in their clinical care to consent for treatment of anxiety and mood disorders.

B.10 Psychology

- Cognitive or intellectual assessments to assist with a better understanding of a person's abilities. Having this information can help the team tailor interventions.

- Assessment of other relevant psychosocial factors to inform a coherent psychological formulation of a person's needs which leads to the design or a comprehensive psychosocial intervention package.

- Consultation to help integrate biopsychosocial information from the various professional assessments into complex formulations.

- Adapting and presenting psycho-education in a format that is accessible to the various recipients of the information (client, family, staff groups).

- Treatment: a wide range of psychological interventions are available. These include group, family and individual counselling/therapy from a variety of perspectives including cognitive-behavioural therapy, psychodynamic therapy, family systems therapy, solution-focussed interventions, narrative therapy and play therapy. See also behavioural therapy.

- Supporting other services to adapt approaches so that they become more meaningful to the person with intellectual disabilities according to that person's needs.

References

1. Banks, R., Bush, A., Baker, P. *et al.* (2007) Challenging Behaviour: A Unified Approach, Royal College of Psychiatrists, British Psychological Society and Royal College of Speech and Language Therapists, London, CR 144. Available at: http://www.rcpsych.ac.uk/files/pdfversion/cr144.pdf.

2. Ball, T., Bush, A. and Emerson, E. (2004) *Psychological Interventions for Severely Challenging Behaviours Shown by People with Learning Disabilities: Clinical Practice Guidelines*, British Psychological Society, Leicester. Available at: http://www.bps.org. uk/downloadfile.cfm?file_uuid=4A51DB4D-306E-1C7F-B697-0FDC56A88DC9& ext=pdf&restricted=true.

Index

References to tables are given in bold type. References in figures are given in italics.

Intellectual Disability Psychiatry: a practical handbook   Angela Hassiotis, Diana Andrea Barron and Ian Hall (eds)
© 2009 John Wiley & Sons, Ltd

carers 117, 209
  assessment of decision-making capacity
    by 39
  communication with professionals 14
  information-sharing 23
  intervention in psychotic illness 80
  psychiatric assessment of mood disorders
    and 59
  see also informants
*Carers at the Heart of 21st-Century Families and
  Communities* 14
Carpenter syndrome 140
catatonia, autism and 96–97
catatonic schizophrenia 72
cerebral palsy 8, 141, 145
  older people 150
challenging behaviour 30–31,
    122–126, 187
  aetiological conditions 116
  assessment
    antecedents, behaviour and
      consequences (ABC) 124
    baseline data 124
    data analysis 125–126
    diagnosis 118–119
    frequency and duration 124–125
    questionnaires 125
  autism spectrum disorder 90
  behaviour therapy 226–227
  chronic 128–129
  concept 115–116
  context and 116–117
  definition 115
  language 117
  management 126–130, 128
    in the community 126–127, 130
    in-patient 130
    medication 129
    positive behaviour support
      127–128
    specialist services 129–130
  mental health crises and 186
  non-verbal communication and 10
  prescription of drugs and 208
  socio-political context 118
  see also offending behaviour
Charles Bonnet syndrome 76
childhood autism 87

children
  autistic spectrum disorder 87, 88
  challenging behaviour 126
  decision-making 48–49
  developmental milestones **22**
Children's Act 1989 49
chlorprozamine 79, 219
cholinesterase inhibitors 161
classification systems 2, 30
  mood and anxiety 56–57
  see also DC-LD; DSM-IV; ICD-10
clinical assessment 261
  assessment tools 34
  behavioural problems 30–31
    offending behaviour 173
  emergency 194–196
  establishing communication 23–25
    discordant information 25
  examination 33–35
  information-gathering 21–22
  insufficient symptoms to make diagnosis 30
  interview setting 22
  mood disorders 57–61
  patient history 32
  presenting problems 28–30
  questioning 26–28
  role of a third person 32–33
  transient symptoms 31
  see also cognitive function assessment;
    diagnosis; interviews
clozapine 78, 204
cocaine 105
  see also substance abuse
cognitive behaviour therapy (CBT) 80, 179,
    205–206, 227–229
  key assumptions **228**
cognitive function
  assessment 158–159
  measurement 35
collateral history 14
communication 2, 16–17
  about medication 203–204, 211–212
  with carers 14
  clinical assessment 23–24
    communication styles 23–25
    questioning 26–28
  context and 12–13
  definition 3–4

dental disease **135**, 141, 144, 188
Department of Health, Michael Report
recommendations 136
dependence syndrome **102**
depressive disorders
cardiovascular disease and 143
challenging behaviour and 119
cognitive behaviour therapy 228
dementia and 160
epilepsy and 142
ICD-10 classification and 254
pharmacological treatments 205, 207
physical health and 138
respiratory disease and 143
deprivation of liberty 46–49
deputies (Mental Capacity Act) 45–46
development
anxiety and 52
history 32
milestones **22**
see also developmental disorders
developmental disorders 29, 120–122
see also development
diabetes **138**
diagnosis 27–30
anxiety and mood disorders 56–57
autism spectrum disorder 89
dementia 156–157
diagnostic overshadowing 28–29, 58,
187–192, 194
emergency 198–199
psychotic illness 68
transient 31
see also clinical assessment; DC-LD;
DSM-IV; ICD-10
diet 56
DiGeorge syndrome 81
digression **24**
diminished responsibility (court plea) 175
Disability Distress Assessment Tool
(DisDAT) 9
disengagement **24**
disorganized schizophrenia 68
diversity 117
DM-ID 56–57
doctors, communication styles 25
Down's syndrome 9, 55, 59–60, 134,
140, 142

Alzheimer's disease and 155–156, 157
cardiovascular disease 143
dementia 160
medication 162
depressive conditions 160
diagnostic overshadowing 189
obesity and 140
older people 150–151
respiratory disease 143
sensory impairment 4
thyroid disease 32
visual impairment 139
drug abuse see substance misuse
drugs (prescribed) see medication
DSM-IV classification system 2, 56
dementia 154–155
psychotic illness 68
duplication of services 246
dysarthria 193–194
dystonia 220

eating disorders
associated physical diagnoses **138**
autism and 94
see also underweight
echolalia, delayed 11
EEG see electroencephalography
elderly people see older people
electrocardiograms (ECG) 79
electroencephalography (EEG) 34, 77
dementia 160
emergencies see mental health crises
emotional regulation
communication and 12–13
see also mood disorders
endocrine conditions 75
environment
impact on communication 12–13
interviews 22
epidemiology, psychotic illness 69
epilepsy 32, 34, 75, **135**, 141–143
alcohol abuse and 110
antipsychotic medication and 79
autism and 97
automatism 175
drug treatments 142, 218
mental health crises and 189
eugenics 239